# STOMA CARE

# STOMA CARE

### TG Balachandar
MS MCh MAMS FRCS (Edin)

Senior Consultant
Department of Surgical Gastroenterology and Proctology
Apollo Hospitals
Greams Road, Chennai, Tamil Nadu, India

*Forewords*

### Dr Pratap C Reddy
**(Padma Bhushan and Padma Vibushan)**

### Steven D Wexner

### Professor M Ahmed Ali
**(Padma Awardee)**

### KS Prasanna Kumar Reddy

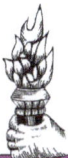

JAYPEE *The Health Sciences Publisher*
New Delhi | London | Panama

**Jaypee Brothers Medical Publishers (P) Ltd**

**Headquarters**
Jaypee Brothers Medical Publishers (P) Ltd.
4838/24, Ansari Road, Daryaganj
New Delhi 110 002, India
Phone: +91-11-43574357
Fax: +91-11-43574314
E-mail: jaypee@jaypeebrothers.com

**Overseas Offices**

JP Medical Ltd.
83, Victoria Street, London
SW1H 0HW (UK)
Phone: +44-20 3170 8910
Fax: +44(0)20 3008 6180
E-mail: info@jpmedpub.com

Jaypee-Highlights Medical Publishers Inc
City of Knowledge, Bld. 235, 2nd Floor, Clayton
Panama City, Panama
Phone: +1 507-301-0496
Fax: +1 507-301-0499
Email: cservice@jphmedical.com

Jaypee Brothers Medical Publishers (P) Ltd.
17/1-B, Babar Road, Block-B, Shyamoli
Mohammadpur, Dhaka-1207
Bangladesh
Mobile: +08801912003485
E-mail: jaypeedhaka@gmail.com

Jaypee Brothers Medical Publishers (P) Ltd.
Bhotahity, Kathmandu, Nepal
Phone: +977-9741283608
E-mail: kathmandu@jaypeebrothers.com

Website: www.jaypeebrothers.com
Website: www.jaypeedigital.com

© 2018, Jaypee Brothers Medical Publishers

*Stoma Care*

*First Edition:* 2018

ISBN: 978-93-5270-487-3

## Dedication

*Dedicated, with affection to all those living with Ostomy and to all those who care for them.*

# FOREWORD

Apollo Hospitals has always been in the forefront in offering quality and affordable medical care to the patients in India and abroad for the past three decades.

This consortium is equally devoted in imparting academics and training to all the students, who are undertaking their courses in many fields of medicines and Dr TG Balachandar, a senior consultant in the department of Surgical Gastroenterology from this institution has rightfully fulfilled this commitment and made the institution proud.

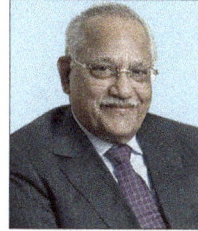

After reading this book, I have learned that this particular "Stoma Care" is very much needed to the patients who undergo such a surgery which requires not only medical care but also a psychosocial approach, for their well-being.

I hope this book *"Stoma Care"* meets the objectives of the GI surgeons, Colorectal surgeons and the Stoma Care Nurses all over India.

I congratulate Dr TG Balachandar for his vision in choosing to publish such a book which has not been addressed so far in India by any author. I hope many consultants will replicate such valuable ideas. I wish him success in all his future endeavors.

**Dr Pratap C Reddy**
(Padma Bhushan and Padma Vibushan)
Founder-Chairman of Apollo Hospitals, India

# FOREWORD

There are a plethora of scholarly volumes which describe in great detail all of the facets of colorectal surgery. Many of these books include information about stomas. The commonality amongst the many textbooks within the field of colorectal surgery, including all of the volumes edited and/or authored by me is that they are written for the healthcare provider generally the surgeon rather than for the patient. I was extremely impressed to read Stoma Care by Dr TG Balachandar, as he has produced a much needed comprehensive and readily understandable compendium of stoma care which I am certain will be immediately embraced by patients around the world.

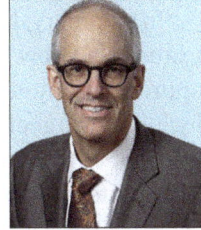

I am delighted that his acknowledgements include my late friend Professor N Rangabashyam in who's memory I had the honor of presenting the first annual Professor N Rangabashyam Memorial Oration during the April 2017 Apollo Hospitals International Rectal Cancer Symposium in Chennai, Tamil Nadu, India. Another acknowledgement was to my friend Dr Venkatesh Munikrishnan who is one of the most energetic, enthusiastic, dedicated, and devoted rising stars in colorectal surgery. Venky organized the Apollo rectal cancer meeting including the Rangabashyam oration. I am sure that he will do more than justice to the memory of N Rangabashyam and make Dr TG Balachandar proud. Lastly, I note that further acknowledgements are quite appropriately directed to Dr Pratap C Reddy and Ms Preetha Reddy who have supported our collaboration amongst Cleveland Clinic Florida, the Apollo Hospitals, University College London Division of Surgery, and Advances in Surgery Channel.

Virtually every one of the 181 pages is ripe with information about a myriad of subjects including the history and evolution of the stoma, overview of the digestive system, and the physiology of the stomas. Dr Balachandar explains to patients the types of stomas as well as the diseases which may require stoma creation. He elegantly describes every type of stoma including urinary diversion. He offers some very salient accurate pointers about stoma creation as well as about pouching systems, application of stoma products, and tips for stoma maintenance. He explains ostomy care, ostomy visitors, and special situations including handicapped Ostomates and pediatric Ostomates. He even devotes significant space within his book to the role of social media for the Ostomate which is a very current and important topic. He describes the problems and potential solutions for patients with stomas traveling in India and abroad, as well as offers a list of ostomy associations which may provide further assistance. He poses frequently asked questions and then provides detailed appropriate answers to those questions in an easy to understand manner.

In summary, I am incredibly impressed at the quality of Dr Balachandar's textbook. I know his labors will be rewarded as this unique resource will be appreciated by stoma therapists, patients, and other healthcare providers including surgeons in practice and surgeons in training. Accordingly, I am honored to write this foreword and look forward to recommending this book to my Ostomate patients, stoma therapists, trainees, and colleagues.

**Steven D Wexner**

MD PhD(Hon) FACS FRCS FRCS(Ed) FRCSI(Hon)

Director
Digestive Disease Center
Chair
Department of Colorectal Surgery
Cleveland Clinic Florida
Weston, Florida, USA

# FOREWORD

One of the greatest happiness for a teacher is when his student excels in his profession and earns many laurels. Dr TG Balachandar is one example. Knowing him for last 40 years, I am not surprised by his achievements. He is always committed to his work and his patients. The present book is an example of one such involvement.

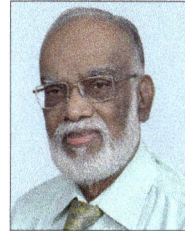

The moment, the possibility of a stoma is revealed to the patients, they are shocked and even refuse surgery. But by sympathetic and kind approach and informing them of the latest facility of Stoma Care, we can alleviate their apprehension.

Many of my patients long years after surgery, have thanked me for my guidance and are comfortable living with the Stoma.

This book will be helpful to all the young colorectal surgeons in day-to-day practice. The historical aspect of the present day Stoma Care is very informative and interesting. I wish Dr TG Balachandar, a grand success of his book *"Stoma Care"*.

**Professor M Ahmed Ali**

MS MCh DSc (Hon Causa)

**(Padma Awardee)**

Former Professor of Surgical Gastroenterology
Madras Medical College
Chennai, Tamil Nadu, India

# FOREWORD

Dr TG Balachandar is known to me for nearly two decades. Soon after GI surgery department was started at Apollo Main Hospital, Chennai, I applied for National Board programmes in Minimal Access Surgery and GI surgery. When I was looking for Faculty who are both good at clinical and academic work, Dr TG Balachandar came to my mind. I requested our Chairman to consider taking him as faculty for GI surgical department which he readily agreed. He has been doing excellent work and he is instrumental for the success rate of our Surgical Gastro Postgraduate programme. This brought laurels to the centre as one of the best and sought after centres for Teaching and training.

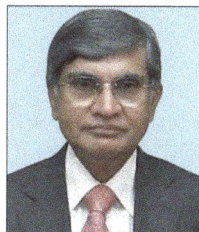

It was a pleasant surprise to see the book *Stoma Care* authored by Dr TG Balachandar and my memories went down the lane during my training years in UK, as stoma (ostomy) was one of the common surgeries performed at that time. It is the only book authored by an Indian author.

The book starts with the Evolution, Anatomy, Physiology, Indications and Complications related to stoma.

The book also details how to live with stoma and about various stoma products available in the market. Very salient feature is preoperative counselling and postoperative reassurance. This is very important as stoma is an unnatural opening in the body, which is a difficult task to accept. The book also details about temporary or permanent stoma. He also mentions the role of a stoma care nurse who teaches and guides people who are not familiar.

Lastly, this book is a valuable addition to all the medical Libraries, postgraduates in General and GI surgery. Good book for reference for General, GI and colorectal surgeons. The unique aspect of this book is simple language and multiple illustrations for medical, stoma care nurses and patients to understand.

Hearty congratulations,

**KS Prasanna Kumar Reddy**
MB FRCS (Eng, Edin, Glas) DSc FACG Dip Lap Surg (Fr)
Senior Consultant (HOD)
Department of Surgical Gastroenterology and
Minimal Access Surgery
Apollo Main Hospital, Chennai
Professor Dr MGR Medical University
Chennai, Tamil Nadu, India

# PREFACE

As a practising gastrointestinal (GI) surgeon for the past four decades, I could not find a book dedicated to the subject of Stoma care wholly serving to the needs of GI surgeons, colorectal surgeons, surgical oncologists and ET nurses and to the Ostomates.

Hence it was my dream to publish a book which has all the information needed for surgeons, ET nurses and Ostomates.

It was found by research that there are a range of physical and psychological problems that patients may experience following surgery which results in the creation of stoma.

Recognition of their problems resulted in the establishment of Stoma care nurses who developed a high degree of knowledge of expertise, which enabled them to meet the specific needs of this patient group.

The Stoma Care has developed during the past 3-4 decades from primitive care to modern management due to feedback from the stoma patients, with the resultant development of stoma care offered by surgeons, ET nurses and WCON.

I believe that caring for the patients who are undergoing surgery and learning to live with a bowel and urinary stoma is both exciting and challenging. It is exciting because each person reacts to their situation and implications for their life and sense of themselves differently. These differences give us the opportunity to work flexibly and creatively with each patient and their family.

Many surgeons and nurses have very little opportunity to develop their experience in the care of stoma patients because they are often small in number. But over the past two decades, the number of stoma patients has increased remarkably, and hence there is a crucial need to offer them quality care right from the beginning of planning of stoma up to the maintenance of established stoma.

There is a growing need for stoma care, as the number of surgeries performed to create a stoma either permanent or temporary or a urinary stoma has considerably increased due to performance of this kind of surgeries by GI surgeons, Surgical oncologists, General surgeons, Colorectal surgeons and surgeons operating on emergency.

But then most of the surgeries are carried in a tertiary hospital or in a specialised unit dedicated to GI surgical unit. There is a lack of expertise available among the surgeons and nurses working in a community hospital who also need to be educated in the creation and maintenance of stoma.

These problems are further compounded in our country when patients who come from remote areas are left without any help and availability of stoma services.

Whichever model exists within a specific area, the essential issue is that, expertise has to meet the needs of the patient, preoperatively, during their hospital stay and once they return home.

Hence this book is written to assist the healthcare professionals, who are caring for ostomates – before, immediately after stoma forming surgery and in the long term.

This book "Stoma Care" is divided into 27 chapters to highlight the issues related in Stoma surgery and care for surgeons from the basics to advancements. This book also outlines the nuances of stoma care to ET nurses and WCON.

At last it is also written to all the Ostomates, the information necessary from the beginning of creation of stoma up to the long term care including the problems faced by the ostomates both physically and physiologically.

I hope with the abled guidance of my teachers I have brought in such a book which may help the stoma nurses and GI surgeons.

**TG Balachandar**

# ACKNOWLEDGMENTS

The concept of ostomy care originated in ward 10, Government General Hospital, Chennai as "Stoma care clinic" in the year1983 for the first time in South India by late Prof. N Rangabashyam who was a pioneer in GI surgery.

I would like to thank all the people who helped me while writing this book.

My heartfelt thanks first goes to late Prof. N Rangabashyam, who appreciated my work and enthusiasm and advised me to write this book, which is necessary to educate the Surgeons, ET Nurses and Ostomates.

I whole heartedly thank our beloved Chairman Dr Pratap C Reddy and our Vice Chairman Ms Preetha Reddy for inspiring and supporting me at the Apollo Hospitals Chennai, to start the DNB Surgical Gastroenterology programme.

I extend my sincere thanks to my colleague Dr KS Prasanna Kumar Reddy, Senior Consultant, Department of Surgical Gastroenterology who was instrumental in starting the DNB Surgical Gastroenterology programme at Apollo Hospitals, Chennai. He has guided and encouraged me in all my academic endeavours.

My special thanks are due to my Mentor and Guru Prof. M Ahmed Ali a senior Surgical Gastroenterologist who always encouraged me to write this book. I also take this opportunity to thank my teachers Prof. RP Shanmugam and Prof. R Surendran who were my role models.

It is my duty to pen my respects to Ms C Saroja who has pioneered in the field of Stoma care in South India and to Ms Syamala Devi and Ms D Selvi—the pillars of "Ostomy Care" Chennai.

I appreciate and cherish my professional duties during my tenure at the Government General Hospital and Stanley Hospital in the Deptartment of Surgical Gastroenterology with Dr D Kannan, Dr P Ravichandran, Dr R Jeswanth, Dr S Rajendran and Dr O Naganathbabu.

I would also like to thank all my colleagues in the Department of Surgical Gastroenterology, Apollo Hospitals, Greams Road, Chennai—especially Dr Venkatesh Munikrishnan, Colorectal surgeon who was instrumental in the promotion and launch of this book. My special thanks to all my Postgraduates of DNB Surgical Gastroenterology for being my inspiration to be a teacher since 2012.

Dr Sudeepta Kumar Swain deserves a special mention for being a constant support in all my endeavours.

I thank all the ET nurses and managers of Ostomy Care group, Tamil Nadu for having magnanimously contributed their experience about the recent trends in Ostomy care and their issues in Indian scenario.

I am indebted to all my patients from whom I still continue to learn.

I wish to thank my wife and children who always supported and encouraged me in publishing this book.

# CONTENTS

1. Introduction     1

2. History and Evolution of Stoma Care     3
   - Stoma Surgery Prior to the 19th Century   *4*
   - Stoma Surgery in the 20th Century   *4*
   - Loop Stomas   *7*
   - Stoma Appliances Prior to the 20th Century   *8*
   - Stoma Appliances in the 20th Century   *8*
   - Historical Stoma Appliances   *10*
   - Development of Ostomy Care in India   *13*
   - Development of Ostomy Care in Tamil Nadu   *14*

3. Overview of Digestive System     16

4. Physiology of Stoma     18
   - Normal Jejunal and Ileal Absorption   *18*
   - Physiology of Stoma   *19*
   - Colostomy   *22*

5. Types of Stoma     26
   - "One" or "Two" Stomas?   *26*
   - General Indications   *27*
   - Gastrointestinal Function   *30*

6. Classification of Stomas     41
   - Conditions Involving the Colon   *41*
   - Conditions Involving the Urinary System   *43*
   - Conditions that may Require Surgery Involving a Stoma   *43*

7. Disease Condition that may Require Surgery Involving Stoma     44
   - Congenital Disease Conditions   *44*
   - Acquired Condition   *45*
   - Colorectal Malignancy   *47*
   - Obstructive Disease Condition   *47*

8. Conditions that may Require Urinary Diversion 50
   - Other Abnormalities of the Urinary Tract 52
   - Urinary Diversions 52
   - Ileal Conduit 53

9. Principles of Stoma Creation and Selecting the Stoma Site 55
   - Where will the Stoma be Placed? 57
   - Stoma Site Selection 59

10. Pediatric Stoma Care 64
    - Conditions that Necessitate a Stoma 65
    - Specific Aspects of Stoma Care 68

11. Pouching System Procedures 71
    - Types of Pouching Systems 71

12. Application of Stoma Products 77
    - Application of One-Piece Fecal Pouch 77

13. Surgical Principles of Stoma 83
    - Temporary Stomas 83
    - Methods of Stoma Construction 83
    - Ostomy Closure and Time 96

14. Role of Enterostomal Nurse 97
    - Preoperative Considerations 97
    - Preoperative Counseling 99
    - Postoperative Role 100
    - Appliances 102
    - Psychological Support 105
    - Diet 106
    - Foods to Avoid 107
    - Lifestyle Modifications of Patients with Ostomy 107
    - Day-to-Day Activity 110
    - Sex and Intimacy 114

15. Tips for Maintenance of Stoma 116
    - Colostomy Irrigation 116
    - Criteria for Irrigation 116
    - Principles of Colostomy Irrigation 117

16. **Patient Related Problems in Stoma** 121
    - Fundamentals of Patient Care *123*

17. **Educating the Stoma Patient** 126
    - Teaching and Counseling for Self-Care *126*
    - Bathing *126*
    - Clothing *126*
    - Fecal Diversions *127*
    - Discharge Planning *127*
    - Ostomate Bill of Rights *127*

18. **Complications of Stoma** 129
    - Complications *129*
    - Stomal Necrosis *131*
    - Retraction *131*
    - Peristomal Skin Irritation *132*
    - Parastomal Abscess, Ulcer, and Fistula *134*
    - Parastomal Hernia *135*
    - Stricture *137*
    - Caput Medusa *138*
    - Mucosal Implants *140*
    - Stomal Prolapse *140*
    - Bleeding and Peristomal Varices *141*
    - Recurrence of Disease *142*
    - Diversion Colitis *142*
    - Diarrhoea *142*
    - Constipation *142*
    - Partial or Incomplete Diversion *142*
    - Trauma *142*
    - Tips for Prevention, Early Deduction and Management of Simple Complications *143*

19. **Teaching Ostomy Care to Nursing Students** 145
    - Planning and Teaching of Ostomy to Student Nurses *145*

20. **Role of Ostomy Visitor** 147
    - The Objectives of Ostomy Visitor *147*
    - The Ostomy Visitor should Understand *148*

21. **Challenges Faced by Handicapped Ostomates**                                150
    - Mental Illness    *150*
    - Visual Illness    *150*
    - Motor Sensory Illness    *150*
    - Role of WOCN and ET Nurse    *151*

22. **Ostomy and Social Media**                                152
    - Facebook    *152*
    - Twitter    *152*
    - Youtube    *153*
    - Websites Offering Stoma Care    *153*

23. **Ostomy Supplies and Agencies in Ostomy Care**                                154

24. **Ostomy Associations in India and Abroad**                                155
    - Ostomy Association of India (OAI)    *155*
    - Ostomates India    *155*
    - Ostomy Service    *155*
    - United Ostomy Association of America (UOAA)    *155*
    - International Ostomy Association (IOA)    *156*
    - Colostomy Association    *156*
    - Australian Council of Stoma Associations Inc    *156*
    - Wound, Ostomy and Continence Nurses Society (WOCN)    *156*
    - Gold Coast Ostomy Association (GCOA)    *156*
    - The Danish Ostomy Association COPA    *157*

25. **Amazing Ostomates**                                158

26. **Frequently Asked Questions**                                162
    - Commonly Asked Questions    *162*

27. **Glossary of Terms**                                172

*Index*                                *183*

# Introduction

According to the available literature, it is estimated that 450,000 people in US currently have a Stoma and 120,000 new surgeries are performed each year.

The United Ostomy Association estimates that slightly more than 500,000 Americans have some type of Stoma. In UK, there are around 130,000 Ostomates.

In India each year, more than a 100, 000 people undergo surgery in which Faecal or Urinary Stoma is made. Majority of the patients who are living with Stoma is due to the treatment given for colorectal cancer. However Stoma forming surgery may be undertaken for other benign conditions like Ulcerative colitis, Crohn's disease, Diverticulitis or complications with Bowels function and genetically predisposed bowel diseases.

In India, every year the incidence of colorectal cancer is increasing in number, but the number of ostomy cases are not much, especially it has been witnessed that in the past 2 decades there is a steady increase in the temporary stomas and a fall in the permanent Stomas which is due to the revolution in the surgical management of Colorectal cancer by Minimal invasive surgery and advancement in the chemoradiation techniques, where in sphincter saving surgery have increased simultaneously with a covering Ileostomy as a temporary measure.

In India there are 300,000 registered Ostomates besides roughly the same number of unregistered Ostomates. On an average about 10,000 Ostomy surgeries are carried out, of which 1/3 may be temporary Ostomies.

In Tamil Nadu, approximately 3000 Ostomy surgeries are happening every year with 70% as temporary and 30% as permanent Stoma. 5% of the total group is Paediatrics. Average age group falls between 40 and 60 of which 40% are females and 60% are males.

In earlier years, the stoma was not envisioned or created by the surgeons but by the forces of nature. For example, the result of a strangulated hernia in those individuals, fortunate enough to survive or those who survive with abdominal wounds with visceral injury live with a permanent enterocutaneous fistula as a Stoma.

But in the modern era, Stoma forming surgery has revolutionised in to a purposeful creation of an opening on the surface of the abdomen which can be well maintained by the patient. These people live normal lives and some of them even enter in to a very challenging professional life.

Advancements in Stoma surgery and Ostomy management systems have given a new ray of hope that, Ostomates can also lead an active and normal life.

## ■ BIBLIOGRAPHY

1.  Diseases of the Colon and Rectum; Centennial Articles in colon and rectal surgeon; Intestinal stomas; 200 years of digging Peter A Cataldo MD. From the Medical Center Hospital, Fletcher Allen Health Care, Burlington, Vermont. https://link.springer.com/article/10.1007/BF02237118
2.  Intestinal Stomas Principles, Techniques and Management second edition, revised and expanded; History of stomas–Peter Cataldo.
3.  Late Stomal complications https://www.ncbi.nlm.nih.gov/pmc/articles/PMC2780194/
4.  Living with an Ostomy in India-Securicare http://www.securicaremedical.co.uk/blog/living-with-an-ostomy-in-india

# History and Evolution of Stoma Care

The history of stomas has its beginnings in Biblical times, but the first purposeful creation of a stoma occurred slightly more than 200 years ago. In a relatively short time, from many of the great pioneers in surgery and enterostomal therapy, the stoma has evolved from a hastily constructed, foul-smelling, and unsightly artificial anus covered with only moss and leaves and held in place with a crude leather strap to an odorless, barely noticeable, and often continent opening that may require no device what so-ever.

One of the earliest accounts of the treatment of traumatic abdominal wounds is found in ancient Hindu writings, Sushruta (600 B.C) advocated the closing of traumatic intestinal wounds with the pincers of black ants, followed by emolument washings and reintroduction of the intestines into the abdominal cavity.

In 1757 Lorenz Heister (1683-1758), after observing the spontaneous formation of stomas following abdominal trauma, recommended exteriorization of the injured intestine. He wrote "that the lips of the intestines so wounded, would sometimes quite unexpectedly adhere to the wound of the abdomen; and therefore there seemed no reason why we should not take hints from nature". In response to criticisms related to the inconvenience of exteriorized intestine, Heister said: "It is surely far better to part with one of the conveniences of life than to part with life itself".

In the eighteenth century, Jean Palfin and John Bell, both barber-surgeons, emphasized closing the wound of the abdominal wall while leaving the injured intestines alone, however, grew more popular throughout the eighteenth century. In 1783 Benjamin Bell modified the exteriorization procedure by creating a double- barreled ostomy in order to prevent stomal stenosis.

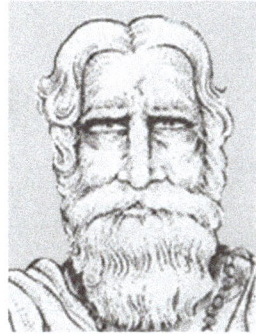

Sushruta Samhita
(Father of Indian surgery)

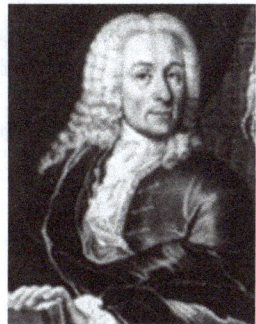

Lorenz Heister
(*Courtesy*: National Library of Medicine, Bethesda, MD)

# ■ STOMA SURGERY PRIOR TO THE 19TH CENTURY

| 55BC-7AD | Celsus | Observations on damage to intestines |
|---|---|---|
| **Key developments in stoma surgery prior to the 19th century** | | |
| 1707 | Lorenz Heister | First recorded stoma surgery |
| 1756 | William Cheselden | Transverse colostomy |
| 1795 | Daguesceau | Fashioned colostomy |
| 1799 | Larrey | Intestine stitched to abdominal wound |

# ■ STOMA SURGERY IN THE 20TH CENTURY

| | Key development in stoma surgery in the 20th century | |
|---|---|---|
| 1913 | John Young Brown | Temporary ileostomy |
| 1923 | Hartmann | End colostomy |

| Key development in stoma surgery in the 20th century | | |
|---|---|---|
| 1943 | Miller | Proctocolectomy and ileostomy |
| 1950 | Bricker | Heal conduit |
| 1952 | <br>Bryan N Brooke | Eversion ileostomy |
| 1969 | <br>Nils G Kock | Internal pouch |
| 1978 | Parks | Preserved anal sphincter |
| 1980 | Mitrofanoff | Internal reservoir for urine |

A surgeon named William Cheselden described his treatment of a patient, Margaret White, had an umbilical hernia from the age of 50, and when she

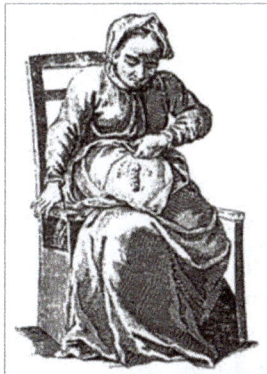

In 1750 Margaret White developed a spontaneous colostomy as a result of a strangulated umbilical hernia (From Devlin HB. Colostomy. Ann R Coll Surg Engl. 1973;52:393-395)

was 73, she had a fit of colic and vomiting which caused the hernia to rupture; it prolapsed and became gangrenous. Cheselden had to remove about 26 inches of bowel and formed a transverse colostomy. He wrote that White recovered and lived for many years and that she was taken out of bed and sat up every day.

In 1710, Alexis Littre of Paris first performed Colostomy through the anterior abdominal wall. Littre's idea remained untested for 66 years, until Pillore, a country surgeon from Rouen, France performed a cecostomy for the treatment of an obstructing rectal cancer.

The colostomy had its true beginning with the surgery of Duret, a naval surgeon at the Military and Marine Hospital at Brest.

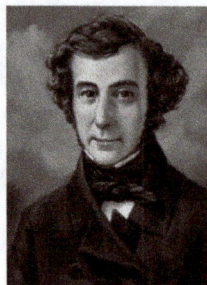

Alexis Littre

In 1793, Duret performed the first successful left iliac colostomy in the treatment of imperforate anus in a 3-day-old infant.

In 1797, Professor Fine, surgeon-in-chief to the Hospital in Geneva, performed the first transverse loop colostomy in a 63-year-old woman suffering from rectal cancer. Through a midline incision, he drew out an inflamed loop of bowel, passed a stitch through its mesentery and sewed it to the skin. The patient's obstruction was relieved and she lived another 3 months.

With the advent of colostomies, it became necessary to create a means for the collection of feces. The first mention of such a collecting device was reported by Daguesceau in 1795. He performed an inguinal colostomy in a farmer who impaled himself on a cart stake while unloading wheat. The farmer, then age 57, survived until the age of 81 and "conveniently collected his feces in a small leather pouch". Daguesceau also performed the first colostomy for the treatment of intractable perianal fistulas. It is interesting to note that the fistulas healed and 2 years later the colostomy spontaneously closed.

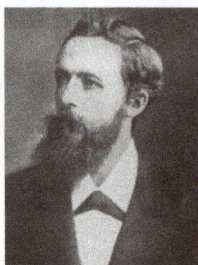

Johann von Mikulicz-Radecki
(*Courtesy*: National Library of Medicine, Bethesda, MD)

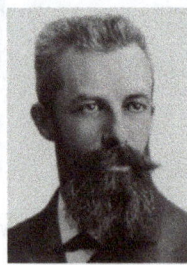

Henir Hartmann
(*Courtesy*: Marvin L Corman, MD)

Technical advances in the creation of ostomies continued throughout the nineteenth century and "resection with exteriorization" became the favored method of colonic resection. At this time, despite the work of Antoine Jobert de Lamballe and Antoine Lembert, primary intestinal anastomosis was considered too risky and therefore was not widely practiced.

However, Mikulicz-Radecki was primarily responsible for the wide acceptance of resection with exteriorization in the surgical community.

Mikulicz recommended his two-stage technique for all resections and anastomoses of the large bowel and for the small bowel when ileus (obstruction) was present.

Hartmann described resection of the sigmoid colon and upper rectum, oversewing of the distal rectal stump and creation of an end descending colostomy and is known as the Hartmann procedure.

## ■ LOOP STOMAS

In 1888, Maydl first suggested the use of an external appliance to support a loop stoma and to facilitate creation of a spur.

In the 1960s the glass rod was replaced by rubber tubing sewn to the abdominal skin, which facilitated the placement of an Ostomy pouch.

Bamn in Germany in 1879 performed a diverting ileostomy in the treatment of an obstructing right colon cancer.

In 1952, Brooke described the classic technique of primary eversion and maturation of the ileostomy, which eliminated ileoserositis and stomal dysfunction.

In 1969, Kock described the creation of an ileal reservoir drained by a tiny stoma brought through the rectus muscle. This method, however, did not lead to complete continence. Therefore, in 1972, he added a nipple valve of intussuscepted ileum.

In 1961, Turnbull opened the first school of enterostomal therapy because of increasing demand for trained enterostomal therapists. Only people with stomas were accepted as students. But many were also trained nurses.

The Ostomy Association of Los Angeles (OALA) began in 1956 as the Ileostomy Association of Los Angeles (IALA) serving the Greater Los Angeles area.

In 1960, fifteen Ostomy support groups from around the country began talking about forming National group. A meeting was held in 1962 leading to the formation of the United Ostomy Association (UOA). The first UOA convention was held in Los Angeles in 1963.

In 1976, Annelise Eidner, a nurse working in the proctology department at the University Hospital Erlangen, Germany, attended the Enterostomal Therapists Nursing Education Program (ETNEP) at the "Rupert Tumbull

School of Enterostomal Therapy", Cleveland clinic, USA. She attended at the suggestion of Dr. Thoflolph Hager, who had just returned from training visit with Dr. Tumbull.

The training of nurse Eidner led to the origin of an Enterostomal therapy that marked the first enterostomal therapy course in the world.

### ■ STOMA APPLIANCES PRIOR TO THE 20TH CENTURY

| Key developments in stoma appliances prior to the 20th century | | |
|---|---|---|
| 1707 | Heister | Tins, silver pipes, cloths |
| 1795 | Daguesceau | Leather drawstring bag |
| 19th century | ---- | Pads, absorbent dressings, binders |

### ■ STOMA APPLIANCES IN THE 20TH CENTURY (FIGS. 2.1 TO 2.6)

| Key developments in stoma appliances in the 20th century | |
|---|---|
| 1910 | Heavy surgical belts with plastic cups |
| 1930s | Thick heavy rubber bags |
| 1944 | Koenig-Rutzen bag |
| 1960s | • Thin odour proof disposable plastic bags<br>• Karaya gum<br>• Hydrocolloid skin barriers<br>• Stoma Care Nurses appointed |
| 1980s | • Plug system<br>• Toilet - flushable colostomy bags |

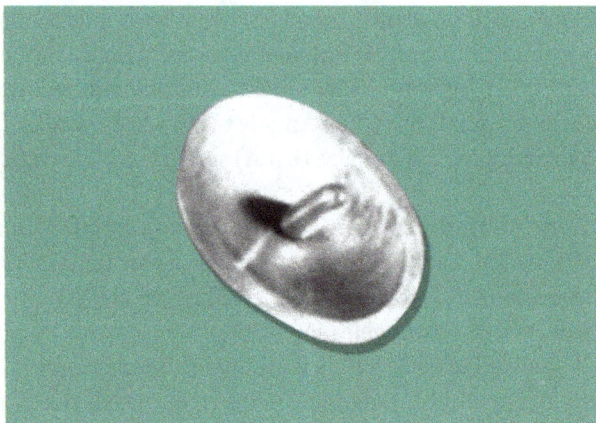

**Fig. 2.1:** Back view of metal colostomy plug, dating from 1920s

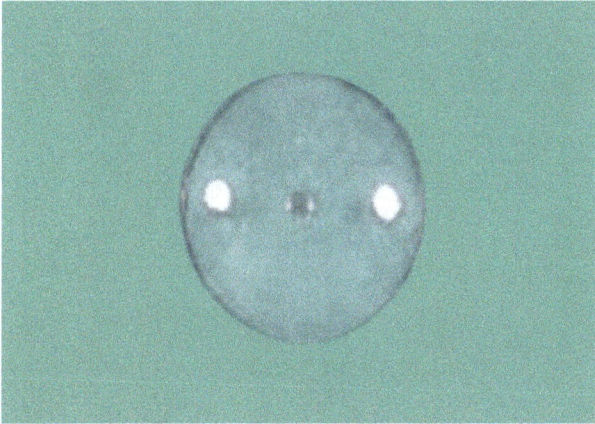

**Fig. 2.2:** A 1930s perspex cup held pads of waddling strapped over a colostomy

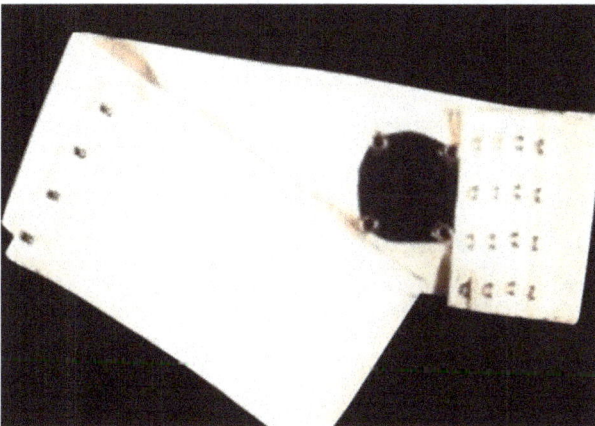

**Fig. 2.3:** Very early two piece showing a corset and base plate

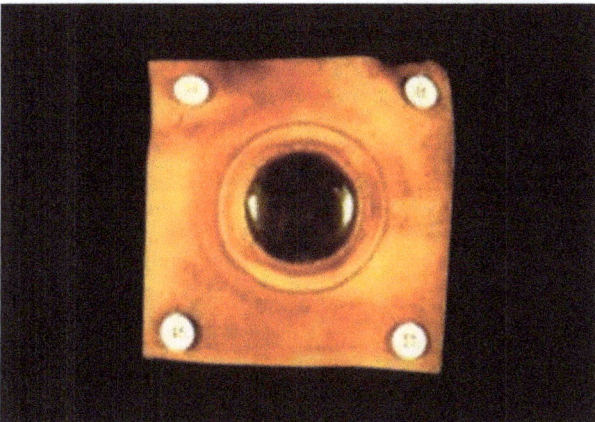

**Fig. 2.4:** Front view of a base plate used as a two-piece

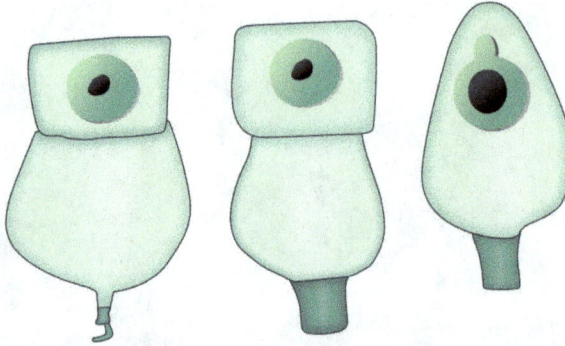

**Fig. 2.5:** Toilet-flushable pouches

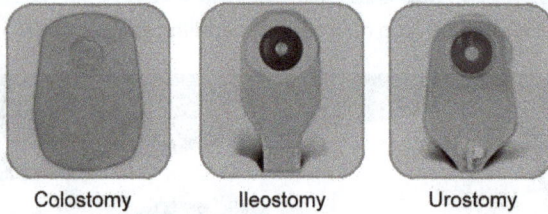

Colostomy     Ileostomy     Urostomy

**Fig. 2.6:** Examples of ostomy pouches

## ■ HISTORICAL STOMA APPLIANCES

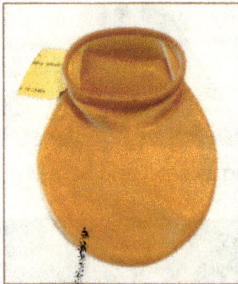

This is an ancient non-drainable stoma pouch made of rubber, which was in vogue before World War II. It was pricey, bulky heavy and complicated to use and needed a belt to the anchor to the abdomen.

Davol product-made out of gum rubber

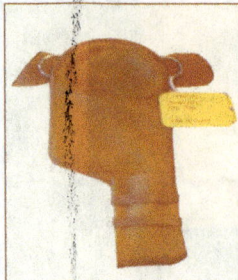

This is a one piece drainable pouch that was in common use. Emptying and cleaning this was a fussy procedure.

First one piece drainable pouch

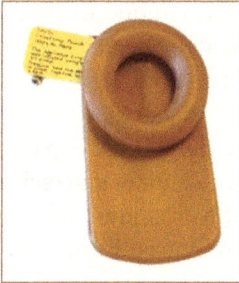

One piece non-drainable deluxe-colostomy pouch with inflatable doughnut that can be adjusted to one's comfort level. They were used even in to the 1960s

Another Davol product with "Comfort" as its only goal

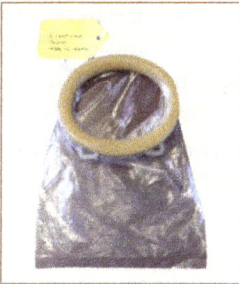

One of the modern pouching systems. A colostomy pouch of 4 parts. A clear plastic bag fastened to the frame by a Gum Rubber ring and a fabric belt to hold the whole thing. It was in use from 1950 to1960s

Stoma pouch made of plastic bag

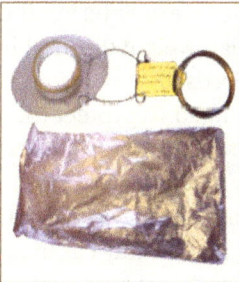

"ABC" colostomy appliance.It was a 6 piece model. A belt, a bag, big Nylon flange, spring wire belt, clear plastic ring with a short spring, another small clear ring between the flange and outer ring

Colostomy appliance made by the Canadian Company of JF Hartz

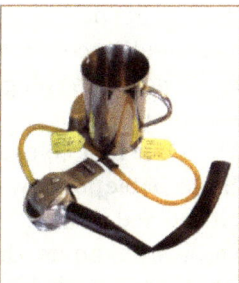

Irrigation system called "The bowman Improved Colostomy Apparatus" made of a stainless steel jug, irrigation cup, rubber catheter and a belt

Appliance specially designed for colostomy irrigation

During the 19th century patients generally relied on pads, absorbent dressings and binders and little had changed at the beginning of this century.

From 1910 onwards some patients were managing their stomas by wearing heavy surgical belts with straps and buckles. The belts, which doubled up as support garments, incorporated in plastic cup over the stoma. The patient would line the cup with cotton wool, lint or gauze dressing which would be changed as necessary. We can only imagine how restrictive and uncomfortable it must have been and how hot and unpleasant in warm weather.

In the early 1940s the first rubber bags were manufactured commercially and it became possible to obtain ileostomy appliances. These first rubber bags were a great improvement on what had been available but they still brought major problems for the wearer. They were large and took a considerable amount of time to fit, as they had to be attached to the skin with adhesives. The adhesives used were often so strong that they caused severe irritation to the skin. The bags were used in rotation and carefully washed out, hung up to dry and turned inside out to be powdered. With frequent use, the bags began to absorb odours and became smelly.

Stoma care for ileostomists took a giant leap forward in 1944 with the introduction of a bag developed in Chicago by an engineering student called Koenig. The Koenig-Kutzen bag was made of thin rubber and was attached to the skin with latex adhesive.

Although rubber bags remained popular were entering the plastic age and people began to see the advantages of lightweight disposable polythenes which did not have to be washed dried and reused.

There was increasing awareness of the need to protect the skin around the stoma. Effectively Karaya gum is collected from trees of Sterculia urens Roxb. in India and its peculiar property is its enormous swelling power. A teaspoonful, in powder form, placed in a glass of water will form a solid jelly-like mass within a few hours. This property made karaya gum powder useful in the textile, cosmetic and food industry and a very common use was for holding dentures in place.

In the 1980s a manufacturer introduced a system described as a plug, which was designed to give the user temporary freedom from wearing a pouch. It is suitable for colostomists with a descending colostomy and with regular bowel frequency. When inserted into the stoma, the plug swells like a tampon and can be kept in situ for up to twelve hours.

Another development during this time was the first colostomy pouch, which was designed to be 'toilet-flushable'. The flushable pouch was welcomed with great enthusiasm by colostomists as it seemed to offer a solution to pouch disposal problems, especially when away from home. Unfortunately a few reports of problems and embarrassment caused by chocked pipes and drains meant that initial enthusiasm waned and patients were reluctant to risk flushing them away. In the early 1990s a company introduced a more successful product which is a colostomy pouch with a toilet disposable liner. The user removes the liner from the outer pouch and flushes it away in the toilet where it biodegrades in the sewage system.

## Modern Appliances

Modern appliances are divided into three main groups: Drainable, Closed and Urostomy. Each of these groups of products is available in one-piece and two-piece versions.

Drainable pouches are used in the immediate postoperative period and where the fecal output is liquid or semi-formed. All ileostomists wear a drainable pouch and some colostomists with a more fluid output need them. They can be emptied via the outlet, which is then sealed with a plastic clip or flexible tie.

Closed pouches are worn by colostomists with well-formed feces and are discarded after use.

Urostomy pouches incorporate a non-return valve to prevent reflux of urine onto the stoma, thus reducing the risk of infection. They have a tap for emptying and can be connected to a drainage system.

One-piece appliances are the most simple to use being lightweight and discreet. The pouch incorporates an adhesive flange to secure it to the skin and after use it is removed and replaced by a new one.

Patients often experience problems because of flatus, or wind, which can create embarrassment by causing their pouches to "balloon". This ballooning can disrupt sleep and can increase the risk of leakage. Closed pouches have long integral charcoal filters, which allow flatus to be released while absorbing any odour. In the late 1990s modern technology has enabled this solution to be available to ileostomists. Some pouches include a filtration system, which allows the filter to remain effective by protecting it from the more fluid fecal output of the ileostomist.

There is a wide range of accessory products available to patients including Pastes, Wafers, Protective rings seals and Wipes, Deodorant sprays.

## ■ DEVELOPMENT OF OSTOMY CARE IN INDIA

The development of ostomy care in India was seen at Tata memorial Hospital (TMH), Mumbai, India. Mrs Anjali Patwardhan, was the 1st trained enterostomal therapist in India in 1975.

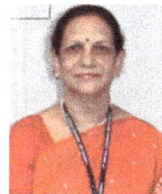

She underwent training on enterostomal therapy under the leadership of Dr Rupert Turn Bull—the colorectal surgeon and Mrs Norma Gill (who was a

Mrs Anjali Patwardhan

rehabilitated Ostomate) who was an enterostomal therapist from Cleveland Clinic, USA.

It was in 1980, enterostomal therapy school was started by Mrs. Anjali Patwardhan under the leadership of Mr Hiralal Narang (founder of enterostomal therapy school).

Mr Hiralal Narang and Ramakant Shah (founder president of Ostomy association of India) were the pioneers to establish the training course at Tata Memorial Hospital, Mumbai.

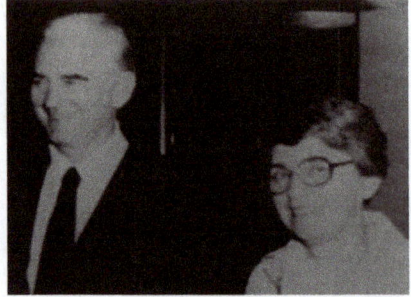
Rupert Turnbull and Norma Gill
(*Courtesy*: WC McGarity, MD)

## ■ DEVELOPMENT OF OSTOMY CARE IN TAMIL NADU

Late Prof N Rangabashyam a renowned surgeon, after obtaining his education and experience from UK, established the Department of Surgical Gastroenterology at the Madras Medical College and Government General Hospital, Chennai, India in 1975.

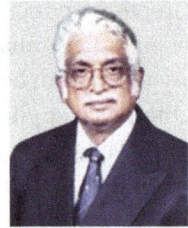
Professor N Rangabashyam

He was the 1st to start the M.ch; course in Surgical Gastroenterology in India and subsequently Nursing Diploma course in Enterostomal therapy.

It was in ward 10, Government. General hospital that he started the "stoma care" clinic in the year 1984 in southern India. He has done a pioneering work in the field of Coloproctology.

Needless to say sister CA Saroja who completed her enterostomal therapy course at Tata Memorial Hospital, Mumbai in 1983, joined the Department of surgical gastroenterology headed by late Professor N Rangabashyam.

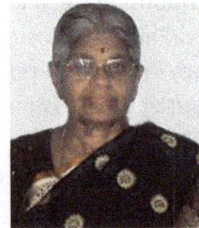
CA Saroja

Sister Saroja had a brilliant academic career and won several awards in surgical nursing and enterostomal therapy. She has published several papers on the subjects like, Ostomates, role of ET and Urostomy care. Inspired by her abilities and dedication in the field of patient care, Prof. N. Rangabashyam appointed Ms. C.A. Saroja as the 1st ET nurse to lead the Stoma clinic of the Department of Surgical Gastroenterology, Government General Hospital, Chennai.

Under the leadership of sister Saroja, several ostomates were attended and educated. She trained many nurses, the principles of enterostomal therapy and many of them are now doing great service in different parts of Tamil Nadu and other states.

Many Ostomates across Tamil Nadu, India are benefitted by able minded nurses trained in Enterostomal therapy under her tutelage.

## ■ BIBLIOGRAPHY

1. Aries L. Colostomy and ileostomy retainer. Int Surg. 1973;58:490.
2. Brown JY. The value of complete physiological rest of the large bowel in the treatment of certain ulcerative and obstructive lesions of this organ. Surg Gynecol Obstet. 1913;16:610-3.
3. Cromar CDL. The evolution of colostomy. Dis Colon Rectum. 1968;11:423-46.
4. First colostomy Stoma Appliances-1900s to Today. http://www.ostomyland.com/ostomyland/lifestyle-guide-chapter-index-2/chapter-21-stoma-appliances-1900s-to-today/
5. Greene HG. Loop colostomy-bar versus rod. Dis Colon Rectum. 1971;14:308-9.
6. Intestinal Stomas by Peter A Cataldo, John M Meckaigan pg. 1-35.
7. Ostomy service - stomacare.co.in

# Overview of Digestive System

To understand how an Ostomy works, it is helpful to know how our digestive system works. Refer the Figure 3.1 below.

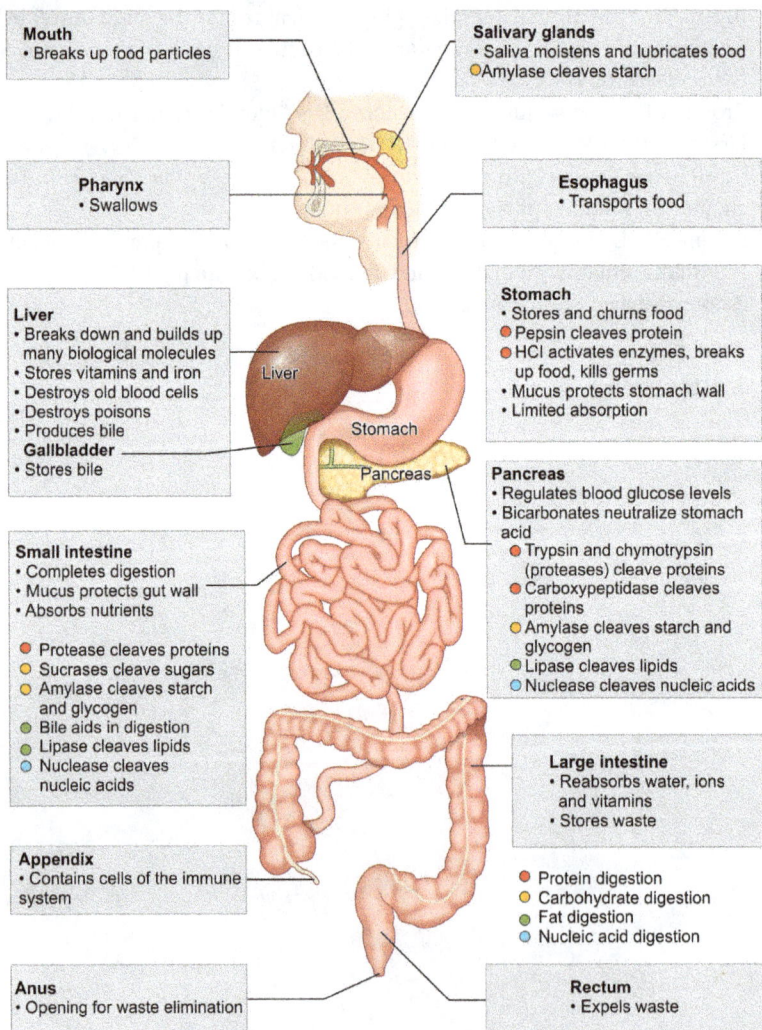

**Mouth**
• Breaks up food particles

**Salivary glands**
• Saliva moistens and lubricates food
• Amylase cleaves starch

**Pharynx**
• Swallows

**Esophagus**
• Transports food

**Liver**
• Breaks down and builds up many biological molecules
• Stores vitamins and iron
• Destroys old blood cells
• Destroys poisons
• Produces bile
**Gallbladder**
• Stores bile

Liver

Stomach

Pancreas

**Stomach**
• Stores and churns food
• Pepsin cleaves protein
• HCl activates enzymes, breaks up food, kills germs
• Mucus protects stomach wall
• Limited absorption

**Pancreas**
• Regulates blood glucose levels
• Bicarbonates neutralize stomach acid
• Trypsin and chymotrypsin (proteases) cleave proteins
• Carboxypeptidase cleaves proteins
• Amylase cleaves starch and glycogen
• Lipase cleaves lipids
• Nuclease cleaves nucleic acids

**Small intestine**
• Completes digestion
• Mucus protects gut wall
• Absorbs nutrients

• Protease cleaves proteins
• Sucrases cleave sugars
• Amylase cleaves starch and glycogen
• Bile aids in digestion
• Lipase cleaves lipids
• Nuclease cleaves nucleic acids

**Large intestine**
• Reabsorbs water, ions and vitamins
• Stores waste

**Appendix**
• Contains cells of the immune system

• Protein digestion
• Carbohydrate digestion
• Fat digestion
• Nucleic acid digestion

**Anus**
• Opening for waste elimination

**Rectum**
• Expels waste

**Fig. 3.1:** Human digestive system—parts and functions
*Picture courtesy:* https://humananatomyly.com/digestive-system-label-and-function/
digestive-system-label-and-function-digestive-system-parts-and-functions-of-human-
human-anatomy-chart-2/

The Human digestive system comprises of digestive organs running from Mouth to the Anus. The food from the mouth enters the Esophagus which acts only as the transporting tube between the Mouth and the Stomach without any role in digestion.

The semi digested food travels down from the Stomach to the Small intestine. The digestive juices produced by Liver and Pancreas act on the semi digested food in the intestine and complete the process of digestion.

The figure given above summarizes the different functions of the different parts of the digestive system.

## ■ BIBLIOGRAPHY

1. Digestive System Overview: Anatomy & Physiology. anatomyandphysiologyi. com/digestive-system-overview/
2. Gastrointestinal System Overview - Medical Art Library. www.medicalartlibrary. com/gastrointestinal-system/
3. Ostomy care and management. John Hopkins medicine -Health Library.
4. Overview of the Digestive System | Anatomy and Physiology. https://opentextbc. ca/anatomyandphysiology/.../23-1-overview-of-the-digestive-syste.

# Physiology of Stoma

## ■ INTRODUCTION

Patients who are subjected to intestinal stoma retain normal physiology with well compensated changes in fluid and electrolyte homeostasis. But sometimes these patients are subjected to variations in the output leading to disturbances in the fluid and electrolyte homeostasis.

Hence, it is necessary for us to understand the normal physiology and systemic response to fecal diversion.

## ■ NORMAL JEJUNAL AND ILEAL ABSORPTION (FIG. 4.1)

Under normal conditions, approximately 90% of nutrients are absorbed within the 1st 150 cm of the small intestine. In the intact Gastrointestinal tract 9–10 liters of endogenous fluid enters the small bowel daily. This fluid

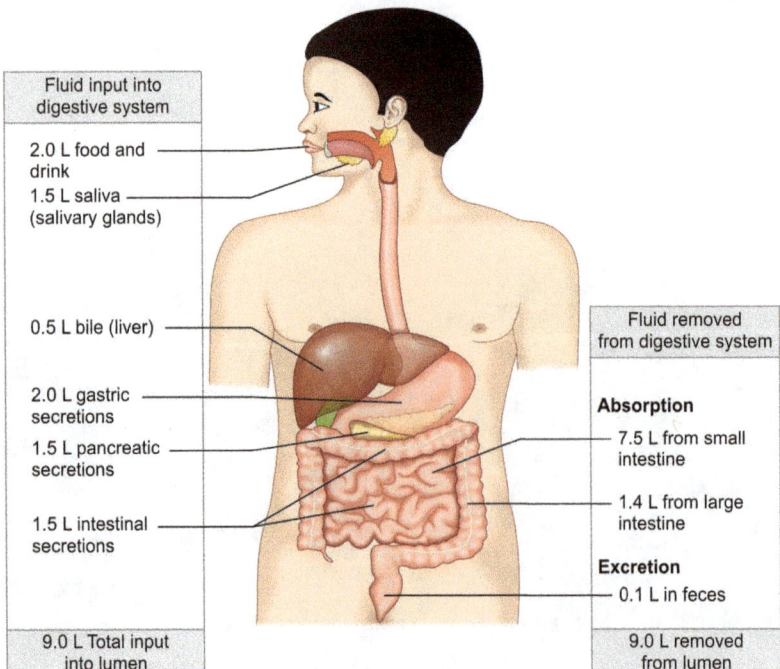

Fluid input into digestive system

2.0 L food and drink
1.5 L saliva (salivary glands)

0.5 L bile (liver)

2.0 L gastric secretions

1.5 L pancreatic secretions

1.5 L intestinal secretions

9.0 L Total input into lumen

Fluid removed from digestive system

**Absorption**
7.5 L from small intestine
1.4 L from large intestine

**Excretion**
0.1 L in feces

9.0 L removed from lumen

**Fig. 4.1:** Gastrointestinal secretions

is composed of Saliva and Bile (approximately 1 liter each) and Gastric and Pancreatic juices (1.5–3 liters combined).

Nearly 6 liters of enteric contents are absorbed in the jejunum and 2.5 liters in the Ileum. This absorptive pattern results in 1.5 liter of content entering the colon daily. 90% of the liquid entering the cecum is absorbed in the colon, leaving approximately 0.1 liter of fluid in the feces.

The differences in absorption within the intestinal segments depend in part on electrolyte transport processes and the permeability of the intercellular spaces.

In the jejunum, Sodium is absorbed actively and moves with bulk flow of water through relatively large mucosal pores. Sodium absorption is enhanced by intraluminal glucose, other actively absorbed monosaccharides, amino acids and bicarbonate ions.

Two main processes mediate the absorption of Sodium and Chloride.

The first is, coupled to the absorption of carbohydrates and amino acids and the second is isotonic sodium chloride absorption. The first occurs primarily in the jejunum, whereas the second occurs principally in the ileum and colon.

Water transport is passive and depends upon osmotic forces. Potassium also moves across the mucosa, following its concentration gradient between lumen and blood modified by a small electric potential of Jejunal mucosa. Bicarbonate disappears rapidly from the lumen by mechanisms that involve active ion absorption & neutralization of bicarbonate by hydrogen ions in chyme.

The ileum absorbs vitamin B12 & Bile salts. Normally the hepatic synthesis of bile salts does not meet the demand for fat digestion. This need is met by Ileal re-absorption of bile salts, which are then recycled into the jejunum. These functions are unique to the segment of the small intestine and have important implications in patients with either ileal disease or resection. Inadequate absorption of bile salts in the ileum alters digestion and absorption of fat in the jejunum and frequently causes diarrhea.

The ileum significantly slows intestinal motility. Intestinal transit studies reveal that markers traverse the first 50% of the small bowel in one-third of the time as the ileum. Thus, ileal resection in turn results in shortened small bowel transit time and increased ileostomy output. Since the motility of the Jejunum is rapid and that of the distal ileum slow, Jejunum resection alone does not result in a faster rate of intestinal transit. In contrast, the remaining bowel has a very rapid transit after ileal resection.

## ▪ PHYSIOLOGY OF STOMA

### Effects of Oral Intake

The influence of diet and fluid intake on the consistency and volume of ileal effluent has been well studied and characterized. Water intake plays virtually no role in determining ileostomy output except that dehydration is associated with decreased outputs and thicker consistency.

## Intestinal Consistency and Erosiveness (Fig. 4.2)

The stool becomes more solid as it progresses through the gastrointestinal tract. A stoma from the colon rather than the small bowel emits stool that is far less injurious to the skin.

Associated with decreased outputs and thicker consistency, Fasting dramatically decreases Ileostomy output between 50 and 100 mL/day. Studies of individual dietary components show that ileostomies respond to the institution of an elemental diet with decreased output and concentration of digestive enzymes and bile acids.

Diets with high fat content have been associated with increase of stomal output to 20% above baseline. Increases in fiber content in excess of 16g/day likewise are reported to increase output by 20–25% and also cause increased stool frequency and flatus. The quantity of sodium in the diet correlates directly with the volume of stomal output without affecting the dry weight of stool. The vast majority of patients, report on maintaining or gaining weight after Ileostomy construction, with tolerance of most food types.

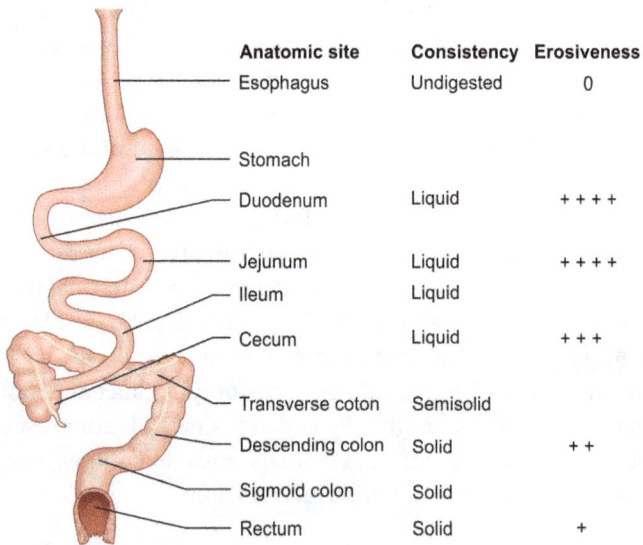

| Anatomic site | Consistency | Erosiveness |
|---|---|---|
| Esophagus | Undigested | 0 |
| Stomach | | |
| Duodenum | Liquid | + + + + |
| Jejunum | Liquid | + + + + |
| Ileum | Liquid | |
| Cecum | Liquid | + + + |
| Transverse coton | Semisolid | |
| Descending colon | Solid | + + |
| Sigmoid colon | Solid | |
| Rectum | Solid | + |

**Fig. 4.2:** Intestinal consistency and erosiveness. The stool becomes more solid as it progresses through the gastrointestinal tract. A stoma from the colon rather than the small bowel emits stool that is far less injurious to the skin
*Source*: From Keighley MRB. Ostomy Management. In: Pemberton JH, ed. Shackelford's Surgery of the Alimentary Tract, 5th ed. Vol. IV. Philadelphia: WB Saunders Co., 2002;305-333.)

## Nutritional Effects

Normal nutrition is the goal and generally also the rule in patients with established ileostomies. As long as terminal ileal resections are limited (less than 100 cm), there are few nutritional consequences. Normally, nutrients are readily absorbed from the small intestine. When malabsorption does occur though, osmotic diarrhea may result and is suggested by malodorous floating stools. Fat malabsorption, from impaired Bile salt absorption of a reduced bile salt pool, is a common cause of osmotic diarrhea. Bile salts may increase outputs either by absorptive inhibition or perhaps by a direct secretory stimulation on the intestinal mucosa. Other disorders of nutrient malabsorption occur with carbohydrates (lactase deficiency) and protein (enterokinase deficiency). Body composition is preserved if patients increase their dietary consumption of fluid, nutritious foodstuffs, and minerals. However, fat losses cannot be compensated for the dietary measures if the terminal ileum has been resected.

In individuals with well-adapted ileostomies, electrolyte, mineral and vitamin deficiencies are uncommon. Intestinal water absorption is controlled by solute transport across the epithelium, with sodium transport being the major determinant of small bowel water absorption. Kramer [II] observed that variations in dietary $Na^+$ do not markedly influence the $Na^+$ content of the stomal effluent. However, chronic systemic water and sodium depletion associated with ileostomy are accompanied by profound changes in urine volume, osmolality and Na+ content.

If dietary sodium is decreased, a diuresis with reduced renal sodium excretion and increased ileal potassium losses occurs, which maintains a normal plasma sodium concentration. Importantly, this renal response may lead to hypovolemia in ileostomates who are already at risk for dehydration because of fixed salt and water losses.

The normal amount of sodium lost in the ileostomy effluent is approximately 60 mEq daily, as compared to 2 to 10 mEq lost in the stool daily in a normal individual. Stomal sodium losses average 1 mEq/hr in the fasting state but increase to 3–4 mEq/hr postprandially. However, symptomatic salt depletion in well-established Ileostomates is rare. Instead, urine output and sodium excretion are decreased because of enhanced renal conservation of salt and water. Hill showed that, despite adaptation, a decreased amount of total body water and exchangeable sodium exists in ileostomy patients compared to healthy persons. This obligatory ileal sodium loss is normally overcome with a standard diet. Importantly, however, the onset of volume depletion is rapid in patients who develop high ileostomy outputs for any reason.

## Bacteriological Environment

The bacterial flora of the ileum after ileostomy is intermediate in nature between small intestine and colon. Gorbach et al. found an 80-fold increase in organisms in the terminal Ileum, furthermore, coliforms were 2500 times more common than in normal ileal fluid. Overall, the ileostomy effluent bacterial count was still considerably less than that of normal feces. Staphylococci, streptococci and fungi were increased in number, while Bacteroides fragilis was rarely found in the ileostomy effluent.

## Systemic Effects

Urinary stone formation is a widely recognized complication of inflammatory bowel diseases, particularly in association with ileal resection. The reported incidence is 3–13% and is related to dehydration and excess sodium losses experienced by patients with ileostomies. The incidence of stone formation in the general population is approximately 4%. Uric acid stones usually make up less than 10% of all stones but 60% of all stones found in patients with ileostomies. Christie et al. found ileostomy and Ileal Pouch Anal Anastomosis (IPAA) patients to have a significantly lowered urinary volume and pH, with increased concentrations of calcium and oxalate. Patients with ileostomies were at increased risk for forming uric acid and calcium stones, while those with IPAA showed only a propensity to form uric acid stones. High-output ileostomies and extensive ileal resection predispose patients to stone formation.

The association between ileostomy construction and increased gall stone formation is controversial. Well-adapted patients excrete bile acids in amounts similar to those excreted by a person with an intact colon. However, with extensive terminal ileal resection or inflammation, the enterohepatic circulation is disrupted. Subsequently, bile acid malabsorption or depletion alters the saturation of bile, promoting precipitation and stone formation. Ritchie found no difference in the number of ileostomy patients who required cholecystectomy compared to those without Ileostomies.

## ■ COLOSTOMY

### General

Approximately 1500–2000 mL of fluid and 120 mEq of Sodium are passed daily from the ileum to the colon. The colon secretes little fluid to add to this volume, rather, the colon stores the fecal content and slowly propels the stool in a caudad direction for eventual evacuation. During the passage of stool from the right to the left colon, absorption is so efficient that less than 200 mL of water and 25 mEq of sodium are expelled daily in the feces. To a lesser extent, the colon absorbs bile acids not absorbed in the terminal ileum. However, ileal resection predisposes the patient to excessive colonic bile acids, which promote secretion of water and electrolytes.

When a colostomy first begins to function, the output is liquid. The liquid steadily increases in volume and is expelled on an irregular basis. After 10–14 days the consistency of the effluent becomes quite viscous. Slowly, a pattern of stool evacuation develops and the stool is expelled on a more predictable basis.

In general, the diet of a patient with a colostomy should be unrestricted. The patient soon recognizes specific foods that increase stomal output or flatulence. As in the case of an ileostomy, high-fiber foods increase fecal weight. If sufficient colonic absorptive surface is preserved proximal to the colostomy, dehydration and electrolyte disturbances are rarely matters of concern.

Medications introduced through the stoma are readily absorbed. The exceptions are enteric-coated or time-release formulas, which may be expelled before adequate absorption has occurred. This situation is more of a problem with proximal colostomies, in which excretion is common.

## Proximal Colostomy

Ileal content that enters the right colon is predominately liquid. The right colon is important for mixing the ileal effluent to facilitate water and electrolyte absorption through uniform exposure of the luminal contents to the mucosal surface. The cecum and the ascending colon store and knead the luminal contents through a series of antiperistaltic annular contractions. The proximal colon is the origin of giant migrating contractions responsible for mass movements of luminal contents distally. Constructing an ascending or proximal transverse colostomy interferes with the storage and mixing of stool and reduces the absorptive capacity of the colon. Hence the output from these stomas is a high-volume liquid effluent with a high sodium concentration. Fecal material is expelled from a right-sided colostomy on frequent and irregular basis, which allows little or no planned control of stomal output. For these and other reasons, right-sided colostomies should be avoided whenever possible.

## Middle Colostomy

The mid colon is responsible for transit and absorption of the luminal contents. The motor activity is characterized by annular contractions that divide the fecal mass and propel it distally and proximally in a to-and-fro fashion. The construction of a distal transverse or descending colostomy increases the length of absorptive surface and allows enhanced colonic mixing of the fecal material. Sodium is actively absorbed, thereby generating osmotic gradients that facilitate passive absorption of water. Hence the effluent from distal transverse and descending colostomies is lower in volume and less liquid than that from proximal colostomies.

## Distal Colostomy

The distal colon functions primarily as a storage area for fecal material until wilful defecation occurs at an appropriate time. Infrequent strong contractions in the distal colon, which are occasionally sensed by the patient, facilitate caudal propagation of fecal material. The consistency of the fecal matter reaching the distal colon is ordinarily semisolid to solid in nature. After construction of an end-sigmoid colostomy, the colonic contents, composed of unabsorbed food products and bacteria, are expelled, usually no more than once or twice a day. Hence regulation of stool elimination from a distal colostomy through the use of irrigation techniques is often possible. Irrigation initiates colonic distention, which stimulates colonic peristalsis and mass contractions and thus facilitates stool evacuation.

Fecal volumes in a sigmoid colostomy approximate the losses from an intact colon. Like the small intestine, the colon adapts to increased fluid losses from the gastrointestinal tract via Aldosterone-mediated fluid and Sodium resorption by the colonic epithelium. Thus fluid and metabolite homeostasis is facilitated by preservation of the colon proximal to the colostomy, with active participation of the colon in the correction of volume and salt depletion.

## ■ CONCLUSION

The small intestine and colon are critical organs that play a central role in maintaining fluid and electrolyte homeostasis. Nearly all patients adapt to the physiological changes caused by the creation of an intestinal stoma provided that there is sufficient healthy proximal intestine. Metabolic disturbances in patients with stomas are often subtle and develop gradually. Careful attention to fluid and electrolyte balance is therefore necessary to preclude complications related to intestinal diversion. Nonetheless, the metabolic consequences of creating an intestinal stoma are minor and by themselves, rarely alter the patient's lifestyle dramatically.

## ■ BIBLIOGRAPHY

1. Brooke BN. Management of ileostomy including its complications. Lancet. 1952;2:102-4.
2. Christie PM, Knight GS, Hill GL. Dis Colon Rectum. 1996;39:50. https://doi.org/10.1007/BF02048269

3. Crile G Jr. Turnbull RB. The mechanism and prevention of ileostomy dysfunction. Ann Surg. 1954;140:459-66.
4. Gorbach, et al. Principles and practice of Surgery for the Colon, Rectum and Anus;Third edition.
5. Hill GL, Millward SF, King RFGJ. Normal ileostomy output: close relation to body size. Br Med J. 1979;2:831-2.
6. Hill GL. Ileostomy: Surgery, Physiology and Management. New York : Grune and Stratton, 1976.
7. Intestinal Stomas - Principles, Techniques and Management; second edition, revised and expanded; Peter A Cataldo, John M Meckaigan; Stoma Physiology; William E. Taylor John H. Pemberton pg.39-51.
8. Keighley MRB. Ostomy Management. In: Pemberton JH (ed). Shackelford's Surgery of the Alimentary Tract, 5th ed. Vol. IV. Philadelphia.

# Types of Stoma

## ■ "ONE" OR "TWO" STOMAS?

When the bowel is divided to remove or bi-pass disease or injury, the surgeon will decide the best procedure for you to aid your recovery (Fig. 5.1, Flowcharts 5.1 and 5.2).

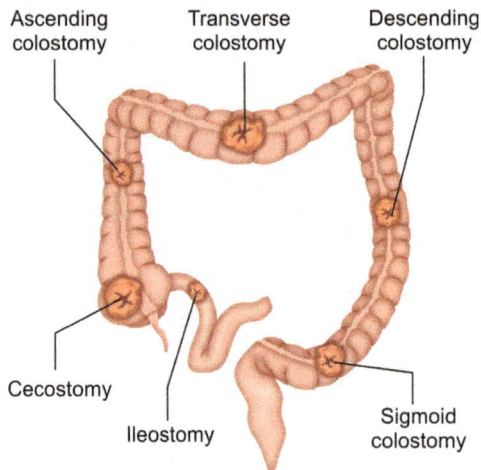

**Fig. 5.1:** Sites of abdominal stomas

**Flowchart 5.1:** Classification of stoma based on the site

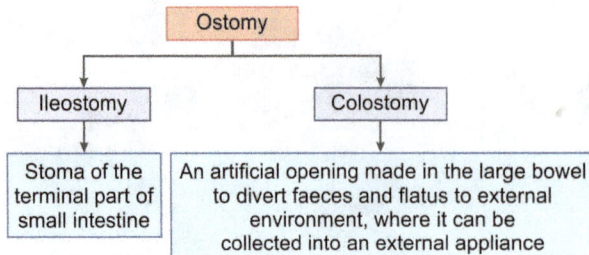

**Flowchart 5.2:** Stoma classification based on anatomical site, type and duration

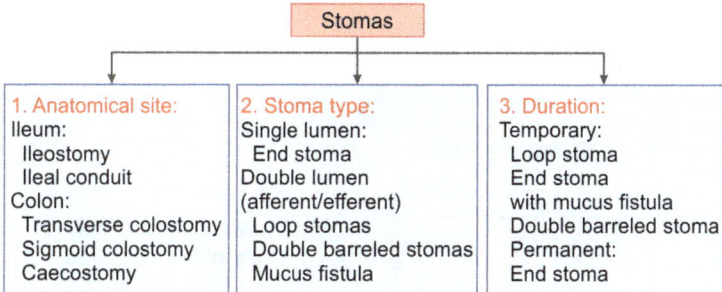

```
                    ┌──────────┐
                    │  Stomas  │
                    └──────────┘
```

| 1. Anatomical site: | 2. Stoma type: | 3. Duration: |
|---|---|---|
| Ileum:<br>  Ileostomy<br>  Ileal conduit<br>Colon:<br>  Transverse colostomy<br>  Sigmoid colostomy<br>  Caecostomy | Single lumen:<br>  End stoma<br>Double lumen<br>(afferent/efferent)<br>  Loop stomas<br>  Double barreled stomas<br>  Mucus fistula | Temporary:<br>  Loop stoma<br>  End stoma<br>  with mucus fistula<br>  Double barreled stoma<br>Permanent:<br>  End stoma |

**Flowchart 5.3:** Classification of stoma based on duration

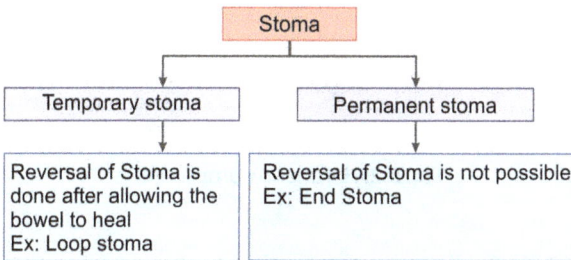

```
                ┌─────────┐
                │  Stoma  │
                └─────────┘
```

| Temporary stoma | Permanent stoma |
|---|---|
| Reversal of Stoma is done after allowing the bowel to heal<br>Ex: Loop stoma | Reversal of Stoma is not possible<br>Ex: End Stoma |

## ▪ GENERAL INDICATIONS (REFER FLOWCHART 5.3)

| Permanent | Temporary |
|---|---|
| • When there is no distal bowel | • To defunction a healing anastomosis |
| • To palliate unresectable distal disease. | • To defunction an intestinal fistula |
| • Incontinence | • To defunction an anastomotic leak |
| • Constipation | • As part of the Hartmann's procedure where an anastomosis is likely to fail |
|  | • In the emergency treatment of obstruction |

- *Hartman's procedure (One stoma)*: Disease is removed; the lower bowel is stitched closed inside you and the end of the upper bowel stitched to your skin as a single stoma (Fig. 5.2). You may experience intermittent urges to pass "stool" from the rectum. This is normal. It is a build-up of mucous in the still healthy rectum. You may sit on the toilet and allow it to pass, but do not strain to push it out!
- *Loop colostomy (One stoma with two openings)*: An incision is made in the skin and the surgeon pulls through it a "loop" of bowel, which is opened but not divided (Figs. 5.3 and 5.4). The loop is prevented from falling back inside by placing a "rod" or "bridge" under the loop until the skin heals

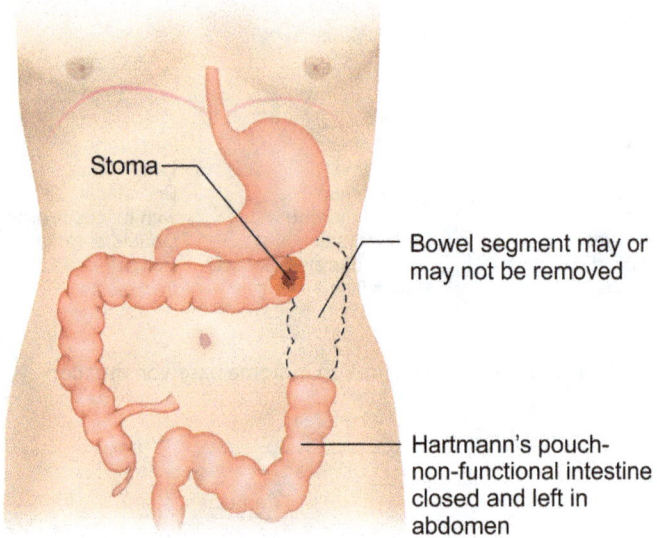

**Fig. 5.2:** Hartmann's procedure

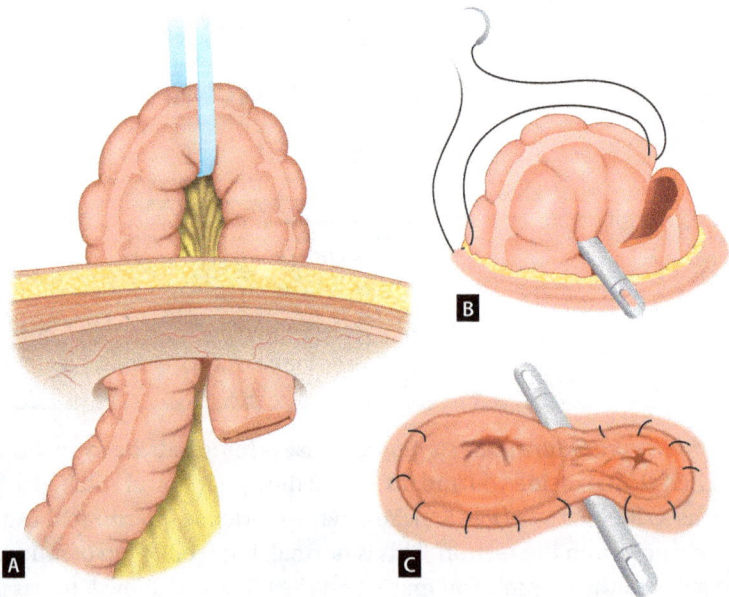

**Figs. 5.3A to C:** Loop end colostomy. (A) A tape or rubber drain is passed through a small hole in the mesentery of the segment of colon to be exteriorized; (B) A plastic rod is placed through the mesenteric opening to support the loop on the skin and is sutured in place; (C) Completed loop colostomy
(*Courtesy*: https://www.researchgate.net/figure/Loop-end-colostomy-A-A-tape-or-rubber-drain-is-passed-through-a-small-hole-in-the_fig7_40688879)

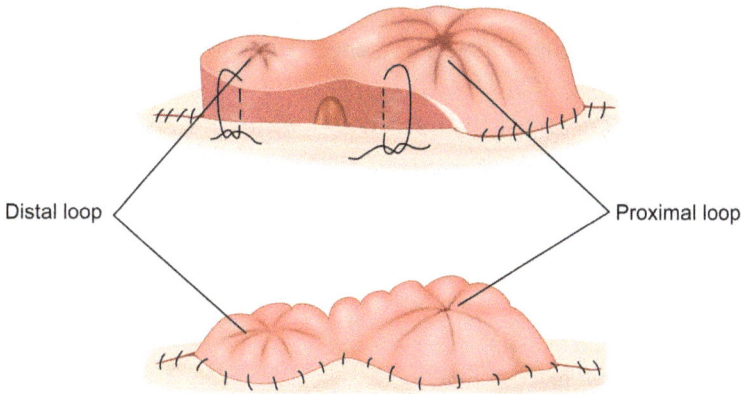

**Fig. 5.4:** Completion of diverting loop colostomy

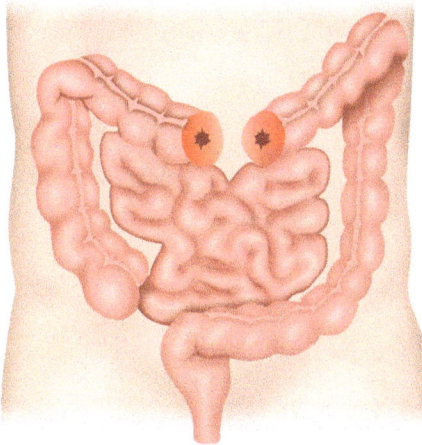

**Fig. 5.5:** Double barrel colostomy

around the stoma in about 6–10 days. The rod will then be removed. This is "one" stoma having "two" actual openings, "Proximal" - from which the stool passes, and "distal" - toward the rectum. You may still experience some stool or mucous discharge from the rectum. This is normal (Fig. 5.4).

- *Double barrel colostomy (Two stomas) (Fig. 5.5)*: An area of disease or injury is removed; the end of the upper bowel is stitched to the skin as a stoma for passing stool. Likewise, the top end of the lower bowel is stitched to the skin as another stoma to allow the lower bowel to decompress or avoid internal inflammation. This second stoma is sometimes called a "mucous fistula" or a "distal-stoma." You may need to wear a pouch on this stoma also, to contain any excessive drainage.

- *Permanent "End" colostomy (One stoma)*: The anus and rectum are removed and the end of the upper bowel is stitched to the skin for the passage of stool.

## Predisposing Diseases Colostomy

- Carcinoma
- Diverticular disease
- Obstruction
- Crohn's disease
- Irradiation damage
- Bowel ischaemia
- Faecal incontinence
- Trauma
- Congenital abnormalities
- Hirschsprungs disease

## ■ GASTROINTESTINAL FUNCTION

### Jejunostomy

Jejunostomy function usually begins within the first 48 hr after surgery (Fig. 5.6). Initially the effluent is watery, clear, and dark green. Because the

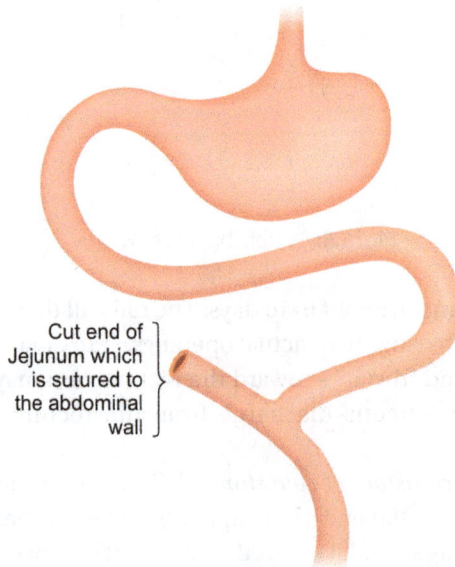

Cut end of Jejunum which is sutured to the abdominal wall

**Fig. 5.6:** Jejunostomy by Maydl's method
(*Courtesy*: Maydl Jejunostomy. Technical and Metabolic Considerations. ES Brintnall, MD; Kate Daum, PhD; NA WOMACK, MD.  https://jamanetwork.com/journals/jamasurgery/article-abstract/550503?redirect=true)

volume of output may approach 2400 ml in 24 hr, the patient should be monitored closely for signs of electrolyte imbalance. Absorption capacity depends on the length and functioning of the proximal bowel. Absorption of nutrients, fluids, and electrolytes may be deficient in the patient with a jejunostomy.

## Ileostomy

An ileostomy generally begins to function within the first 48–72 hr after surgery. The initial effluent is viscous, green, and shiny. An ileostomy created via a laparoscopic approach may begin to function within 24 hrs. Such output does not necessarily indicate return of peristalsis; rather, it may represent the elimination of secretions that have collected in the distal small bowel. Once peristalsis has returned, the patient may enter a period of high volume output known as the adaptation phase. Output during this period exceeds 1000 mL/day and frequently reaches 1500 to 1800 mL/day. The physiological basis for this high-output phase is loss of the colon's absorptive surface coupled with loss of the ileocecal valve. During this period the patient must be monitored closely for signs and symptoms of fluid and electrolyte imbalance. Replacement therapy, which is necessary at this time, can be managed via the intravenous route or with oral electrolyte replacement solutions, depending on the status of bowel function.

Over a period of days to weeks, the proximal small bowel increases fluid absorption and the bowel adapts; gradually the volume of output decreases and the stool thickens to a toothpaste like consistency and is light to medium brown. Initially the output from an ileostomy can vary from 500 to 1500 mL in a 24-hr period. After adaptation, the average output decreases to between 500 and 800 mL daily.

## Ileostomy Predisposing Diseases

### Inflammatory Bowel Disease

- Ulcerative colitis
- Crohn's disease
- Familial polyposis
- Atonic colon
- Defunctioning
  - Obstruction
  - Protect anastomosis
  - Bowel rest.

## Colostomy (Tables 5.1 and 5.2, Figs. 5.7 and 5.8)

The initial output from a colostomy varies, depending on the location of the stoma within the colon. Because the colon absorbs all, but approximately 100 mL of the 1000 mL of contents that passes through the ileocecal valve daily, the output from distal colonic stomas has a thicker consistency and smaller volume than that of proximal colonic stomas.

## Cecostomy

This stoma usually begins to function by postoperative day three. The output may be projectile (because of the close proximity of the ileocecal valve) and initially is liquid. A cecostomy can be either at skin level or tubal. The location, output characteristics, and construction combine to make this a difficult stoma to manage. The tube cecostomy poses a particularly difficult

**Table 5.1:** Comparison of ascending and transaverse colostomy

| Ascending colostomy | Transverse colostomy |
|---|---|
| • *Output*: Liquid to pasty | • Output: mushy, semi formed |
| • *Volume*: Varies | • Volume: varies, could be high |
| • *pH*: Alkaline | • pH: 7.6 |
| • Potential for skin damage | • Potential skin care problems |
| • *Indications*: Obstruction | • Size of stoma causes management problems |
| Tumor or volvulus | • *Indications*: Obstruction |
| • *Location*: Upper right quadrant | Penetrating trauma |
| • *Pouch*: Drainable | RV fistula |
| | Congenital defect |
| | Diverticulitis |
| | • *Location*: Upper quadrant of abdomen |
| | • *Pouch*: Drainable |

**Table 5.2:** Showing list of operative procedures and characteristics of sigmoid colostomy

| List of operative procedures | Sigmoid colostomy |
|---|---|
| • Anterior resection<br>• Abdominoperineal resection<br>• Hartmann's procedure<br>• Subtotal colectomy<br>• Pan-proctocolectomy<br>• Loop Ileostomy ileo-anal Pouch<br>• Ileo-anal anastomosis<br>• Ileal conduit<br>• Colonic conduit | 75% of colostomies in sigmoid area<br>*Output*: Non corrosive, normal, formed stools (semi-solid)<br>Rectum and anus may or may not be removed<br>*Indications*: Carcinoma – (74% of all Ca in Recto sigmoid area)<br>*Pouch*: Drainable<br>        Closed irrigation<br>Skin care problems: Minimal |

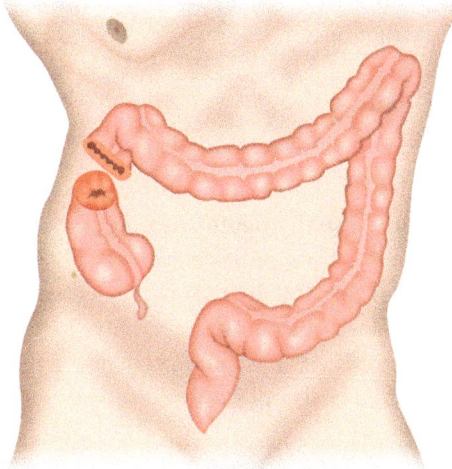

**Fig. 5.7:** Ascending colostomy

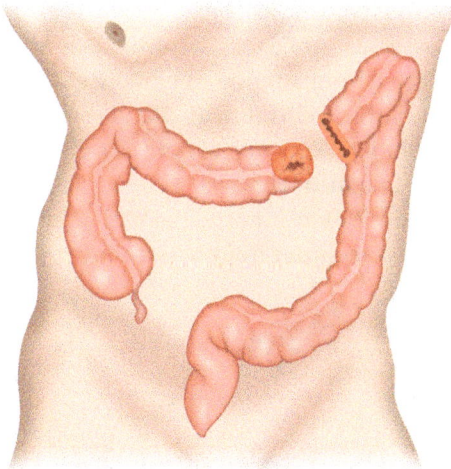

**Fig. 5.8:** Transverse colostomy

management problem because stool tends to flow both through and around the tube. Tube cecostomies also are associated with a greater risk of intra-abdominal spillage.

## Cecostomy

- "blow hole"
- Tube
- Emergency surgery

- Temporary decompression
- Indication—Obstruction
- Pouch—Drainable
- Management nightmare

## Transverse Colostomy

A transverse colostomy usually begins to function on postoperative day 3 or 4. Output, which varies from pasty to soft, usually occurs after meals and at intervals throughout the day. In a loop transverse colostomy, a support device (e.g., rod or bridge) placed during surgery is removed 5-7 days later. The alternative is to construct a fascial bridge at the time of surgery, which obviates the need for a stomal support device.

## Descending or Sigmoid Colostomy (Fig. 5.9)

A descending sigmoid colostomy takes the longest time to regain normal peristalsis and may not begin to function until postoperative day 5. Patients with active bowel sounds who have not passed flatus or stool by postoperative day five should be assessed for factors that would contribute to the delay in return of function (e.g. administration of narcotics). To stimulate function, a 20F soft Foley catheter is well-lubricated and then gently advanced into the stoma. A warm solution of 500 mL of normal saline is instilled via gravity drainage and allowed to return. This procedure initiates a reflex contraction, provides relief of gaseous distension, and maintains peristalsis. Once normal function has returned the output from a descending or sigmoid colostomy

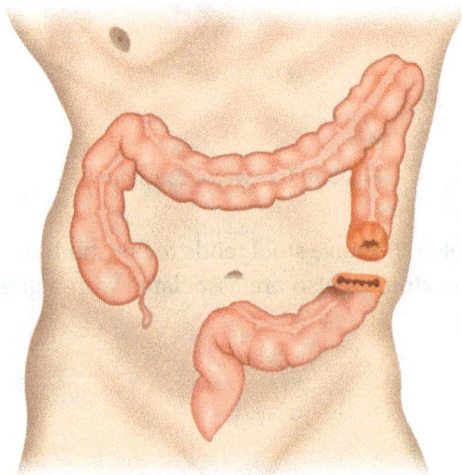

**Fig. 5.9:** Descending colostomy

usually is soft-formed stool. Elimination patterns are generally similar to those of the preoperative period. The amount and consistency of stool from any gastrointestinal stoma is influenced by the amount of bowel resected, the length and condition of the proximal bowel, medications, and diet. Over a period of several months, the remaining bowel increases its absorptive capacity and the effluent decreases in volume and becomes thicker.

## Mucous Fistula (Fig. 5.10)

A mucous fistula is formed at the same time as Ileostomy or Colostomy. It is usually formed during emergency surgery, for ex. in acute colitis or perforation of a bowel with peritoneal contamination, where primary anastomosis is unsafe. In this situation, the proximal limb of the bowel after resection is brought out as functioning stoma and the distal end is brought out and fixed to the abdominal wall, which is called as mucous fistula.

The use of mucous fistula reduces risk of stump dehiscence that occurs in up to 10% of Colostomies for acute colitis. Mucus fistula does not produce mucus but may produce small amounts of feces. The presence of mucous fistula may make subsequent reversal and easier procedure.

## Reversal or Stoma Closure (Fig. 5.11)

Reversal of an Ileostomy or Colostomy involves restoring continuity of the bowel. It should not be attempted before 6 weeks after the original

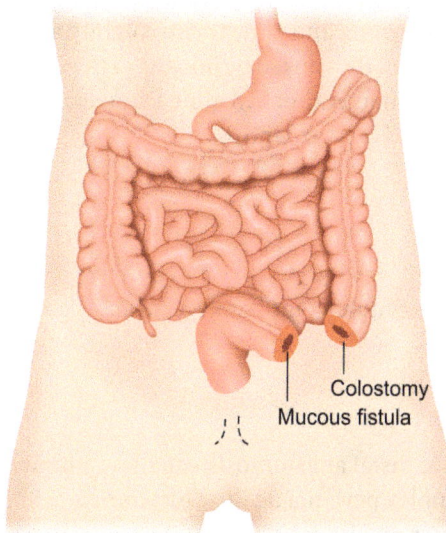

**Fig. 5.10:** Colostomy with mucous fistula

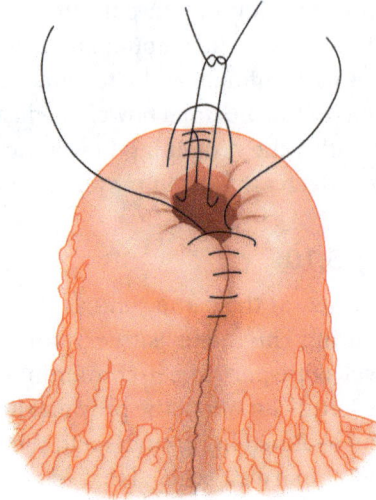

**Fig. 5.11:** Closure of a loop colostomy

operation, when bowel edema has a chance to subside to reduce the risk of complications. If there is a loop or a double barrel Ostomy has been used, then it may be possible to restore continuity without opening the abdomen. There are techniques for closing the bowel with sutures or staples in an end to end or side to side anastomosis.

## Peristomal Skin Protection (Table 5.3)

Urine contains no enzymes and is normally slightly acidic. Therefore, skin damage from urine is usually caused by pooling of the urine on the peristomal skin, which results in maceration. Alkaline urine can damage the skin and cause encrustations and crystal deposits.

## Loop Stoma

### Temporary

Not common in the terminal ileum, transverse and sigmoid colon.

### Loop Colostomy

*Indications:*
- To protect a more distal anastomosis, after low anterior resection.
- Defunction complex perianal fistula procedures.
- Difficult sphincter repairs.
- Fournier's gangrene.

**Table 5.3:** Stoma types and characteristics of discharge

| Type of stoma | Amount | Consistency | pH | Potential to irritate skin |
|---|---|---|---|---|
| | | **Characteristics of discharge** | | |
| Esophagostomy | 1000–1500 mL | Saliva | Slightly acidic | Trends to macerate skin |
| Gastrostomy | Varies | Liquid | 09–15 | Very corrosive |
| Jejunostomy | 1000–1500 mL | Liquid | Acidic | Very corrosive due to enzymes |
| Ileostomy | 1000 mL | Liquid-paste | Alkaline | Very corrosive due to enzymes |
| Cecostomy and ascending colostomy | Varies | Toothpaste consistency | Alkaline | Possible |
| Transverse colostomy | Varies | Mushy-Semi formed | Low potential | |
| Descending and sigmoid colostomy | Varies | Semi-formed | Low potential | |
| Ureterostomy | 1000 mL | Liquid | Slightly acidic | Tends to macerate skin |
| Ileal or colonic conduit | 1000–2000 mL | Liquid with mucus threads | Slightly acidic | Possible |

## How?

A loop of transverse descending or sigmoid colon is brought to anterior abdominal wall, a longitudinal incision is made in the bowel wall and the bowel edges are sutured to the skin.

A purpose made bridge or improvised piece of plastic drain or rubber catheter is used to keep the loop upto the level of the skin whilst healing takes place.

The bridge usually being removed after 7–10 days (reduces risk of retraction and improves faecal diversion )

## When to Close?

Usually after 2–3 months after the primary surgery (distal anastomosis) which is, clinically and radiologically intact.

## Loop Ileostomy

### How?

- The segment of ileum is selected so that it is sufficiently mobile and far enough away from the ileocecal junction that subsequent closure can be easily performed.

- The opening in the abdominal wall needs to be larger than for an end ileostomy.
- A technique using Babcock Forceps can again be used, but an alternative is to make a hole in the mesentery just under the bowel and pass a catheter through this.
- The ends of the catheter are then grasped by forceps passed through the abdominal wall and the stoma brought through by applying tension to the catheter.
- After closing the abdominal wall, the ileum is opened transversely at the level of the skin on the distal non-functioning side.
- To facilitate the identification of this side many surgeons will mark the ileum with diathermy prior to passing it through the abdominal wall. Sutures are placed to evert the ileum in a similar manner to an end ileostomy on the proximal functioning side.
- Everting sutures can also be placed on the distal side to make the whole ileostomy spouted and to facilitate subsequent placement of the ileostomy bag.
- In the emergency situation when the bowel is tending to retract, a rod can be placed under the loop to keep the ileostomy proud of the skin, but in an elective situation such a rod may be omitted and bags are generally easier to fit without one.

## End Stoma
Usually permanent.

### End Colostomy
*Indications:*
- Abdominal perineal resection
- In Hartman's procedure
- Mucous fistula

### How?
An End colostomy is fashioned by bringing the bowel through the abdominal wall through an appropriately - sized split in the rectus muscle (usually 2 finger breadth) and suturing bowel primarily to the skin. (Placement through the rectus abdominis reduce risk of parastomal herniation)

### When to Close?
- Usually permanent
- In Hartman's procedure, 3-4 months later the end colostomy can be reversible after intra-peritoneal tissues recover.

## End Ileostomy

*Indications:*
- Total colostomy for acute severe colitis (ulcerative colitis (or) Crohn's colitis)
- Where ileorectal anastomosis is rarely favored.
- Ileoclic Crohn's disease complicated by intraperitoneal abscess.
- Where immediate ileoileal (or) ileocolic anastomosis is not favored.
- Spontaneous segmental small/large bowel infarction due to thrombo-embolic disease.

### How?
- Because of the liquid contents, it is essential to fashion a Brooke - type evaginated stoma, with a spout 2–3 cm in length, positioned away from skin creases, rib cage and iliac crest
- This is to facilitate application of a well-fitting appliance and avoid skin damage from the effluent (which contains activated digestive enzymes and may be at alkaline PH) and stoma damage from the appliance.

### When to Close?
After the tissue recover, ileorectal, ileoileal, ileocolic anastomosis.

## Mucus Fistula
- Not a stoma
- Is a defunctioned segment of bowel sutured to the skin as a non-functioning stoma.

*Indications:* Emergency setting after subtotal colectomy or segmental resection and end ileostomy, (when the closed distal end of bowel may break down if let inside the abdomen )

- Mucus fistula may be exteriorized at a separate site to an end stoma or suture to end stoma and exteriorized as a double barreled stoma.
- Reversal of double barreled stoma can often be achieved without a laparotomy but they are bulky and difficult to manage.

## Ileal Conduit (Urostomies)
- Stomas producing urine
- Isolated loop of 15–20 cm of ileum with intact blood supply is separated from the rest of the small bowel which is reanastomosed.

  The isolated loop is brought to the skin surface and made into a stoma whilst the other end is anastomosed to the cut ends of the ureters

# ■ BIBLIOGRAPHY

1. A guide to understanding an ostomy-pg.13-30.
2. Clinimed http://www.clinimed.co.uk/Stoma-Care/Stoma-Types.aspx
3. Colostomy Guide –reviewed by Nancy Gutman, RN, CWOCN 2011
4. htpps://www.scribd.com saravanansridharan.
5. http://www.healthcommunities.com/gastrointestinal-surgery/overview-types-ostomy.html
6. Indications and complications of intestinal stomas-Research gate
7. Intestinal Stomas - Principles, Techniques and Management; second edition, revised and expanded; Peter A Cataldo, John M Meckaigan; Stoma Therapy-Ian C Lavery, Paul Erwin-Toth Pg. 67-68.
8. Ostomy overview-Types of Ostomy
9. Types of Ostomies - https://www.hollister.com/brazil/files/care_tips/tips_Types%20of%20Ostomies_1.pdf

# Classification of Stomas

Stomas may be divided into three classifications: input stomas, diverting stomas and output stomas.

1. *Input stomas*: These are usually temporary and facilitate nutrients being put into the gut, e.g. gastrostomy, jejunostomy (Figs. 6.1A and B).
2. *Diverting stomas*: These divert the contents of the gastrointestinal tract away from diseased or damaged gut, e.g. loop ileostomy, and loop colostomy (Figs. 6.2A and B).
3. *Output stomas*: These provide an outlet for the elimination of body waste, usually following excision of an excretory organ, i.e. bladder or bowel, e.g. 'Iliac' colostomy, ileostomy, ileal conduit or urostomy. There are a variety of conditions, which may predispose to surgery involving the creation of a stoma. The most common conditions are described in the chapter (Fig. 6.3).

## ■ CONDITIONS INVOLVING THE COLON

- Ulcerative colitis
- Crohn's disease
- Familial polyposis coli
- Hereditary non-polyposis colorectal cancer (HNPCC)

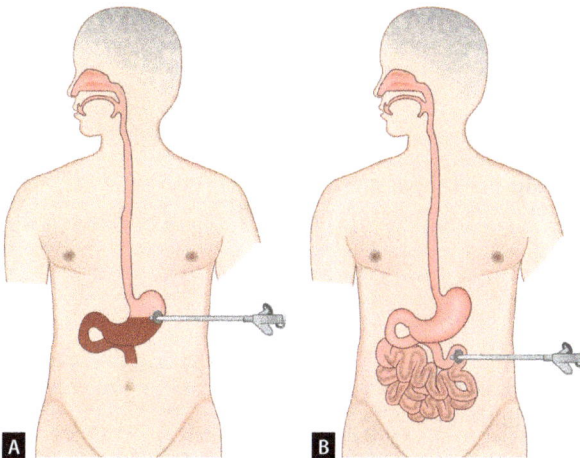

**Figs. 6.1A and B:** Input stomas. PEG tube placement (A). Placement of feeding tube directly into the stomach. PEJ tube placement (B). Placement of feeding tube directly into the jejunum

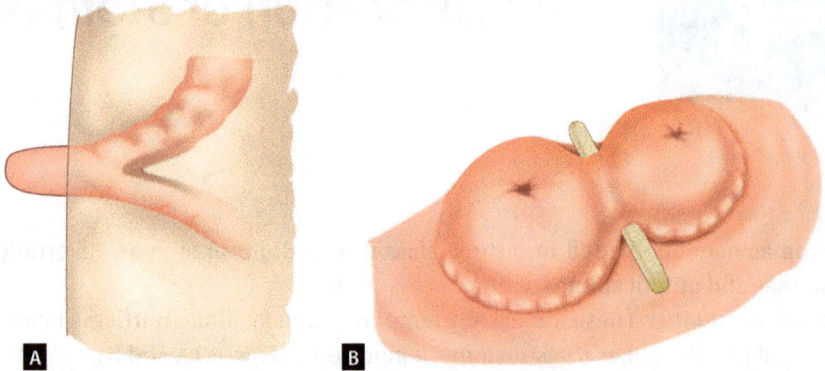

**Figs. 6.2A and B:** Diverting Stomas. (A) Loop Ileostomy: A loop of small intestine pulled out through a cut,then opened up and stitched to the skin to form a stoma. (B) Loop colostomy: Exteriorization of entire loop of colon with proximal and distal limb opening into the common stoma

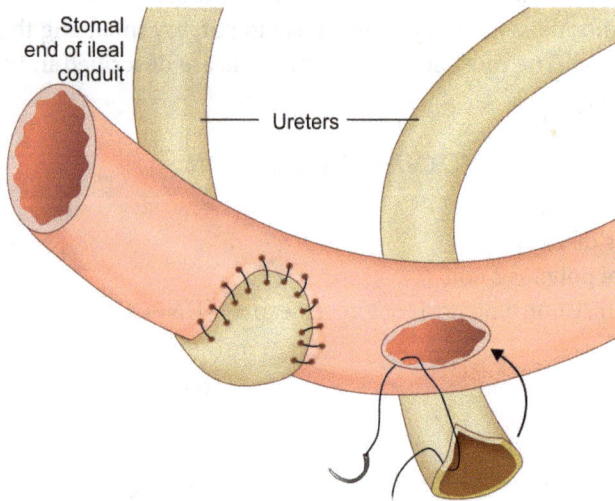

**Fig. 6.3:** Output stoma: Segment of ileum is used for the diversion of urine flow from the ureters

- Colonic cancer
- Rectal cancer
- Diverticular disease
- Colonic obstruction
- Bowel ischemia
- Anorectal incontinence

- Trauma
- Irradiation damage
- Colovaginal/Colovesical fistula

## CONDITIONS INVOLVING THE URINARY SYSTEM

- Bladder cancer
- Contracted bladder
- Urinary incontinence
- Failed uretero-colic anastomosis

## CONDITIONS THAT MAY REQUIRE SURGERY INVOLVING A STOMA

### Pediatric Conditions (Congenital Abnormalities)

- Anorectal anomalies
- Bladder exstrophy
- Cloacal exstrophy
- Spina bifida
- Hirschsprung's disease
- Necrotizing enterocolitis
- Meconium ileus
- Trauma

## BIBLIOGRAPHY

1. Stoma after Ileostomy or Colostomy https://www.betterhealth.vic.gov.au/ health/conditionsandtreatments/stoma-after-ileostomy-or-colostomy
2. Stomas and wound management - Preoperative Considerations and Creation of Normal Ostomies. https://www.ncbi.nlm.nih.gov/pmc/articles/PMC2780193/
3. Stomas of the small and large intestine - http://emedicine.medscape.com/ article/939455-overview

# Disease Condition that may Require Surgery Involving Stoma

## ■ CONGENITAL DISEASE CONDITIONS

### Polyposis (FAP) (Fig. 7.1)

Familial adenomatous polyposis (FAP) is an autosomal dominant disease characterized by multiple adenomatous polyps of the colon and a variety of extracolonic manifestations. They are known to be premalignant and if left untreated, cancer of the colon will almost certainly develop.

### Hereditary Non-polyposis Colorectal Cancer (HNPCC)

An autosomal dominant genetic disorder frequently associated with the incidence of other cancers in distantly related people. The disorder is characterized by the onset of colorectal cancer at an average age of 45 years. This is also associated with the frequent occurrence of other cancers, i.e. uterus, ovaries, stomach and upper urinary tract.

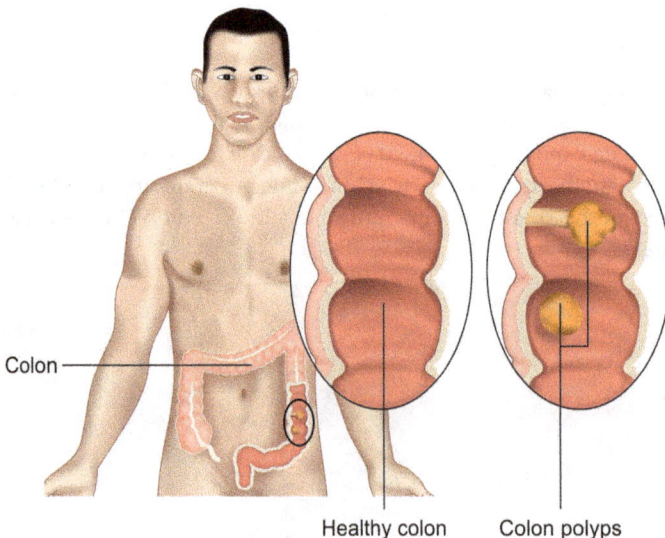

Colon

Healthy colon          Colon polyps

**Fig. 7.1:** Colorectal polyps

## ■ ACQUIRED CONDITION

### Inflammatory Disease Conditions—Nonspecific

#### *Diverticular Disease*

Diverticular disease is a condition in which small pouches (diverticulae) are seen protruding from the bowel wall. It is recognized that patients with such disease have an increased intraluminal pressure.

### Inflammatory Disease Conditions—Specific

#### *Ulcerative Colitis (Figs. 7.2 and 7.3)*

The term "ulcerative colitis" is applied to a disease in which a part or whole of the mucosa of the large bowel becomes diffusely inflamed with a hemorrhagic type of inflammation, which may progress to ulceration.

The symptoms of the disease include diarrhea and the passage of blood and mucus through the rectum. There may be complications of the disease and the patient may become very ill due to anemia, hypoproteinemia and disturbance in the body's fluid and electrolyte balance. During a severe attack, the patient may pass 20 or more stools each day resulting in acute illness and very poor quality of life.

Slightly more women than men are affected in a ratio of 4:3, except in childhood where the sex ratio is reversed. The disease usually takes the form

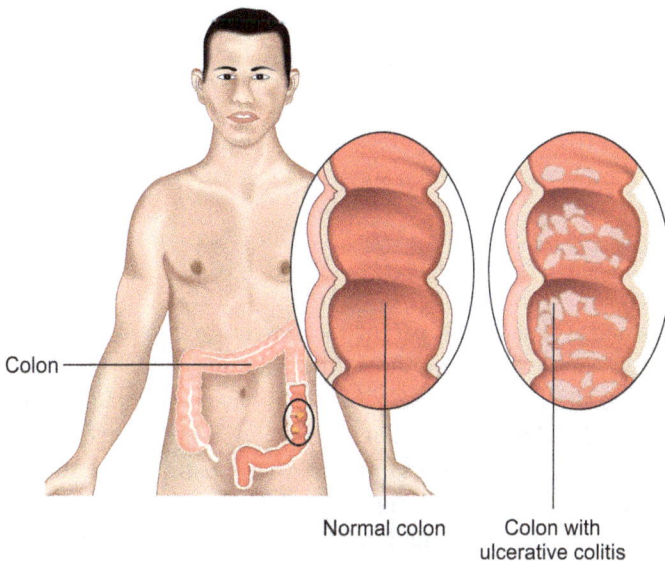

Colon

Normal colon

Colon with ulcerative colitis

**Fig. 7.2:** Inflammation of the inner lining of colon

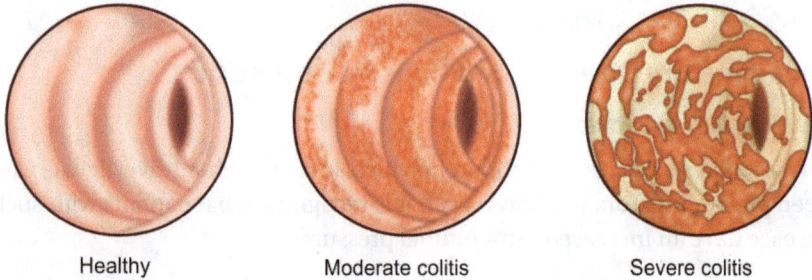

Healthy   Moderate colitis   Severe colitis

**Fig. 7.3:** Stages of ulcerative colitis

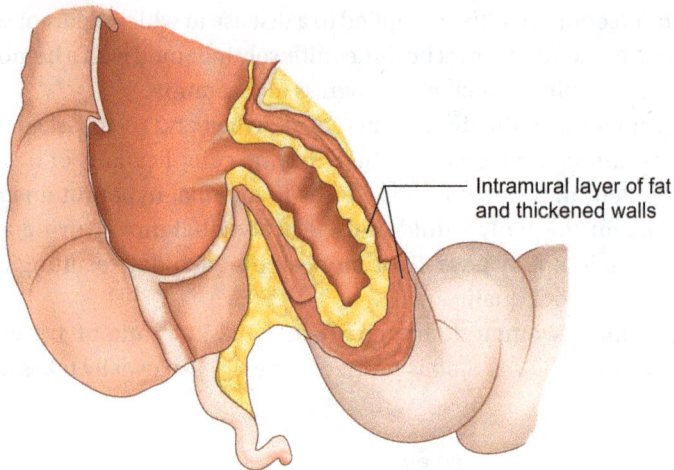

Intramural layer of fat and thickened walls

**Fig. 7.4:** Crohn's disease

of acute exacerbations interspersed with periods of remission. However, there are various situations when surgery to cure the disease is indicated.

## Crohn's Disease (Fig. 7.4)

Crohn's disease is a chronic, progressive, granulomatous, inflammatory disorder, which may affect any part of the alimentary tract from mouth to anus and may be associated with extraintestinal manifestations. The symptoms of the disease are similar to those seen in ulcerative colitis, including diarrhoea, anemia and weight loss. Abdominal pain is symbolic of small bowel disease, as are anal lesions, e.g. Fissures, abscesses and fistulae. Fistula formation, either internal or external, is a feature of the disease possibly caused by leakage via a deep fissure in the bowel wall forming an inflammatory mass in which abscesses develop. These abscesses may burst into an adjacent organ or the exterior of the body. Nutritional support in this situation is of paramount importance. Crohn's disease can affect any part of the alimentary tract and it is characterized by areas of healthy intestine being interspersed with areas of disease, which are known as 'skip lesions'. The quality of life for patients with Crohn's disease can be very poor, due to general ill health, pain, diarrhea, malnutrition and imbalance in the body's fluids and electrolytes.

## COLORECTAL MALIGNANCY

### Carcinoma of the Colon

Carcinoma is a malignant disorder of cell growth arising in epithelial disease. Colorectal cancer is the second most common cause of death from malignancy.

- Hepatic flexure 3%
- Ascending colon 7%
- Transverse colon 4%
- Splenic flexure 3%
- Descending colon 5%
- Sigmoid colon 27%
- Rectum 37%
- Cecum colon 14%

## OBSTRUCTIVE DISEASE CONDITION

### Colonic Obstruction (Fig. 7.5)

Two common causes of colonic obstruction are carcinoma, which has already been discussed and volvulus.

Severe faecal impaction may also result in obstruction.

### Volvulus

A sigmoid volvulus occurs when the gut becomes twisted on its mesenteric axis resulting in obstruction.

### Bowel Ischemia (Fig. 7.6)

If the blood supply to the gastrointestinal tract is compromised, necrosis begins at the innermost layer of the mucosa and spreads outwards; gangrene will ensue within 5-6 hours. The severity and extent of ischemic damage is dependent upon the size of the blocked vessel and the duration of the blockage.

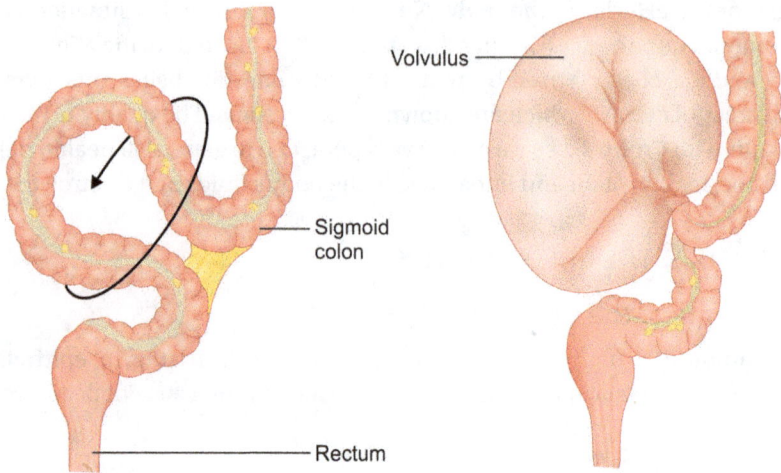

**Fig. 7.5:** Bowel obstruction-Colon

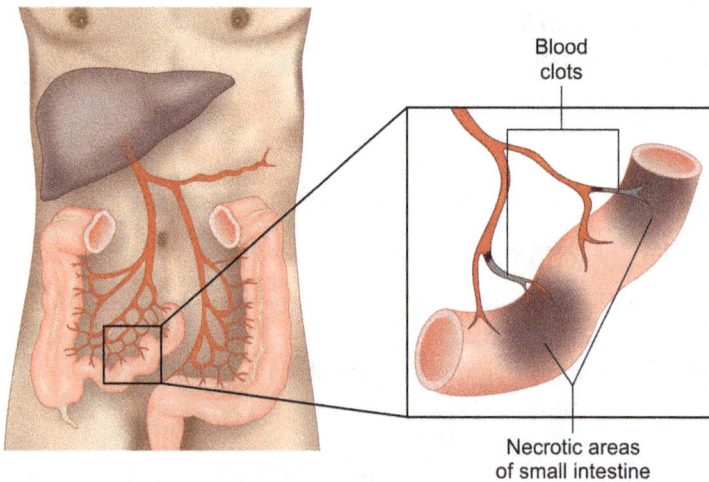

**Fig. 7.6:** Bowel ischemia

*Bowel ischemia can result from a variety of causes, such as*:
- Surgical trauma
- Embolus
- Diseases that produce inflammation of minor arteries resulting in mucosal damage, e.g. systemic lupus erythematosus or rheumatoid arthritis
- Impairment in circulation resulting from cardiovascular disease
- Intestinal obstruction

Bowel ischemia may be considered in two categories: massive necrosis and ischemic colitis.

## Anorectal Incontinence

Continence is dependent upon a balance between fecal consistency and the efficiency of anal sphincter mechanisms. Fluid stools resulting from a disorder of the large bowel such as inflammatory bowel disease or gastroenteritis may not be contained by the anal sphincter resulting in incontinence. Disruption of the anal sphincters may result from:

- Trauma, e.g. impalement injury or obstetric accident.
- Impaired efficiency, e.g. in cases of rectal proplapse or anal neoplasm preventing the anal canal flattening.
- Muscular disorders, e.g. impairment of smooth and striated muscle function.
- Congenital anorectal anomalies.

Many of these conditions are treated by surgical sphincter repair but if this is unsuccessful, the patient may enjoy a much improved quality of life following the fashioning of a proximal diverting colostomy. The treatment of established anorectal incontinence depends upon the cause and severity of the disorder.

## Trauma

Trauma or injury to the abdomen may result in perforation of the intestine. This condition may be seen following road traffic accidents, industrial injury, and stabbing or bullet wounds. Surgery is usually undertaken to defunction the bowel, since leakage of feces must be stopped as a priority. A temporary stoma proximal to the injury is usually created prior to closing the perforation. If the injury involves the small intestine, then resection and primary anastomosis may be performed.

## Irradiation Damage

The bowel is recognized as being sensitive to irradiation. Most cases of rectal damage due to irradiation are associated with the treatment of gynecological or bladder cancer. The symptoms of such damage are usually diarrhea and abdominal cramps in the early stages, but later complications can occur such as stricture, ulceration with fistulae formation, hemorrhage or necrosis.

## ■ BIBLIOGRAPHY

1. Ostomy over view-care of the patient with an ostomy.
2. Stoma Care. Reasons for Stomas discussed in Stoma Care. https://patient.info/in/doctor/stoma-care

# Conditions that may Require Urinary Diversion

*Urinary conduit* is constructed most often after removal of the urinary bladder for invasive cancer.

It is also used for the management of:

- Severe obstruction in urinary tract
- Spina bifida
- Ectopia vesicae or myelomeningocele
- Neurogenic bladder
- Spinal cord trauma

The incidence of surgery for the congenital and traumatic condition is decreasing as on today as other devices of bladder control are in vogue (Fig. 8.1).

It is always better to have a combined team of Urologist and a surgeon familiar with stoma surgery, where in the Urologist carries the primary operation of cystectomy, construction of urinary conduit, Ureterointestinal anastomosis followed by the construction of stoma and restoration of intestinal continuity done by the stoma surgeon.

A well vascularised segment of intestine is necessary to fashion a urinary conduit which later on is to be connected to urinary tract to allow easy flow of urine through the abdominal wall through a stoma constructed exactly like an ileostomy (Figs. 8.2 and 8.3).

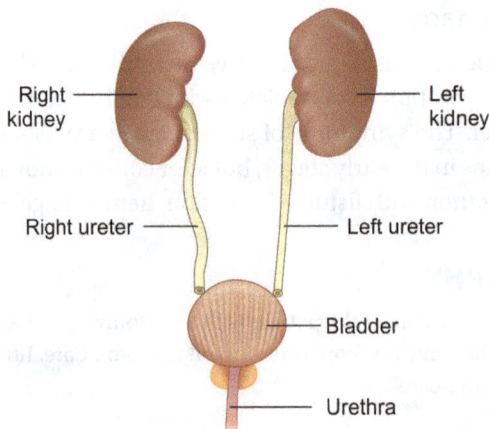

Right kidney — Left kidney

Right ureter — Left ureter

Bladder

Urethra

**Fig. 8.1:** Normal urinary system

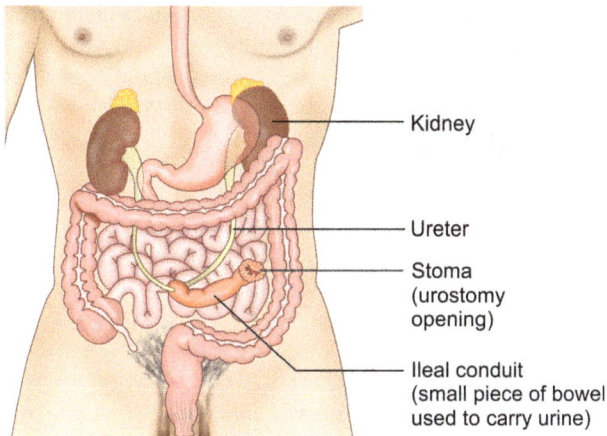

**Fig. 8.2:** Urinary diversion

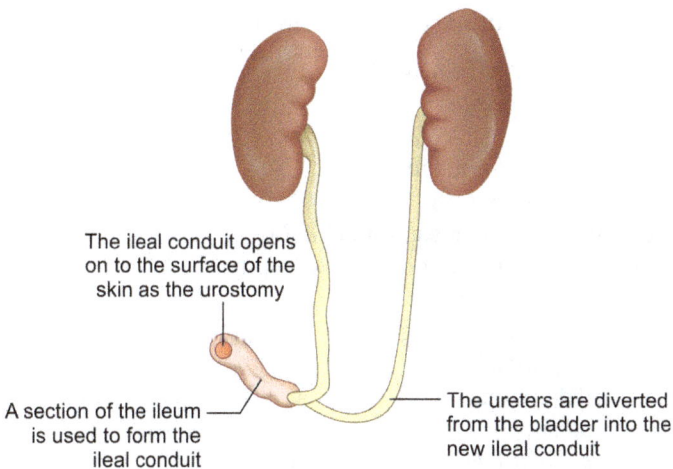

The ileal conduit opens on to the surface of the skin as the urostomy

A section of the ileum is used to form the ileal conduit

The ureters are diverted from the bladder into the new ileal conduit

**Fig. 8.3:** Urinary diversion-ileal conduit

The basic principles of construction of a urinary stoma involve the isolation of a segment of intestine with its mesenteric blood supply and enough mobility to allow the distal end to be used as a stoma and the proximal end to serve as the site for ureteral implantation.

*The following guidelines are to be observed while constructing a urinal stoma*:

- It is important to maintain isoperistaltic direction of the intestine
- The conduit should not be made of irradiated bowel
- There should be proper construction of the stoma otherwise it may lead to stasis of urine resulting in reflex and damage to the proximal tract.

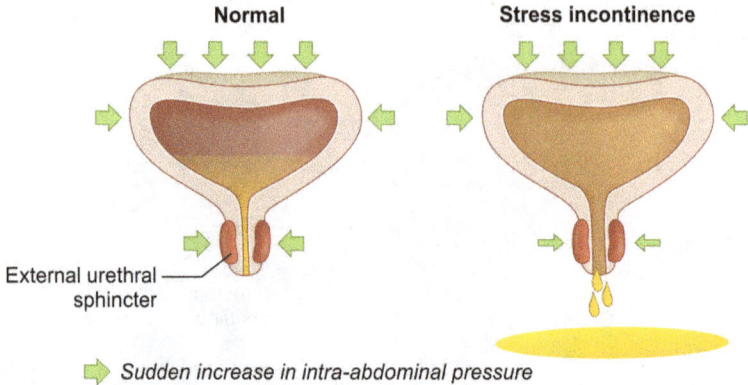

Fig. 8.4: Stress incontinence

Pediatric conditions, such as: Bladder exstrophy; Cloacal exstrophy; Fistulae; and Neurogenic bladder as a result of Spina bifida. Other conditions that may predispose to urinary diversion are as follows:

*Urinary diversion may be indicated if:*
- *The bladder is dangerous*
  - Malignancy
  - Risk of repeated renal infection
- *The bladder is useless*
  - Neurogenic bladder, e.g. spina bifida.
  - Congenital abnormalities, e.g. exstrophy.
- *The bladder is a nuisance*
  - Severe incontinence (Fig. 8.4).
- *The bladder is painful*
  - Interstitial cystitis.
  - Tuberculosis.
- *There is failure of uretero-colic anastomosis*
  - Becomes dangerous because of infection or metabolic complications
  - Leads to incontinence per rectum.

## ◼ OTHER ABNORMALITIES OF THE URINARY TRACT

Urethral-vaginal confluence or cloaca in which there is also recto-vaginal fistula resulting in a single perineal opening leads to urinary incontinence requiring diversion.

## ◼ URINARY DIVERSIONS

### Predisposing Diseases
- Cancer of bladder
- Cancer
- Spinal cord injury

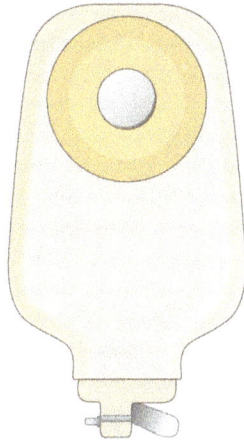

**Fig. 8.5:** Urostomy pouch

- Neurogenic bladder
- Congenital abnormality
- Spina bifida
- Exstrophy of bladder
- Urinary incontinence

## Urinary Diversions

- Ileal conduit (*see* Fig. 8.3)
- Colonic conduit
- Unilateral/bilateral ureterostomy
- Transureteroureterostomy
- Vesicostomy

## Use of Pouch with Urinary Stoma

Issues that must be addressed in regard to applying a pouch to a urinary stoma include peristomal skin protection, pouching options and modifications required for applying a pouch to a stoma with stents in place. Use of an extended-wear barrier will help prevent undermining of the pouch seal and protect the peristomal skin (Fig. 8.5).

### ■ ILEAL CONDUIT

- Most common urinary stoma
- *Output*: 1,500 mL to 2000 mL
- Liquid with mucus
- *pH*: Acidic
- Potential for skin damage and maceration

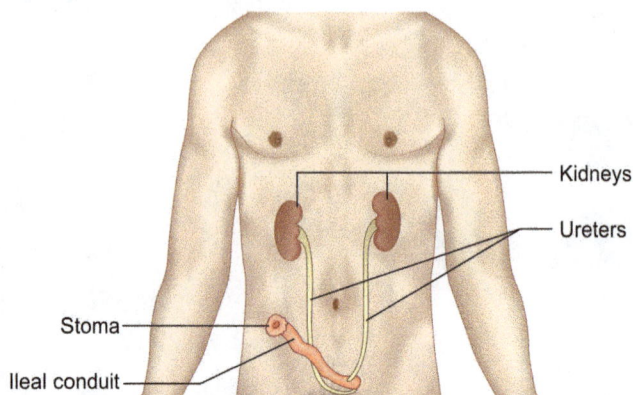

**Fig. 8.6:** Ileal conduit stoma creation

## Location

Right lower quadrant (Fig. 8.6)

## Pouch

Urostomy

## ■ BIBLIOGRAPHY

1. Bricker EM. Bladder substitution after pelvic evisceration. Sug Clin North Am. 1950;30:1151.
2. Ganesan T, Khadra MH, Wallis J, et al. Vitamin B12 malabsorption following bladder reconstruction or diversion with bowel segments. Aust Nz J Surg. 2002;72(7):479-82.
3. Golimbo M. Morales P. Jejunal conduits: Technique and complications. J Urol. 1987;113:787.
4. Intestinal Stomas by Peter A Cataldo, John M Meckaigan.
5. Medical School, Chicago, Illinois, USA. pp. 215-52.
6. Methods of Urinary Diversion—Jeffrey A Stern and Daniel P Dalton, Northwestern University.
7. Wallace DM. Ureteric diversion using a conduit : Asimplified technique. Br J Urol. 1966;38:527.

# Principles of Stoma Creation and Selecting the Stoma Site

The first step in the construction of enterocutaneous stoma is the selection of appropriate site. Stomas should be located within the rectus muscle; if the stoma is brought outside the rectus muscle, the incidence of Parastomal hernia is very high (Fig. 9.1).

> Stoma site marking (to be done with a marker) is not done properly due to lack of availability of stoma nurse at the institution

The objective of stoma construction is to provide an anatomically stable opening allowing placement of an ostomy management system that will maintain a seal of stool and gas for 4–7 days.

If every abdomen were flat, muscular, and unscarred, placement of the stoma would not be a major problem (Flowcharts 9.1 to 9.3).

In reality, many patients have a protuberant abdomen and lax musculature. Often they have incision lines that were placed in different directions and have created creases and weak muscles from neurovascular interruption. Under these circumstances the time taken to plan the site for a stoma is crucial because it can minimize the number of postoperative problems. Siting of the stoma is done with the patient awake.

An ostomy management system or a specially prepared disk of the same dimensions as the system, is used. The patient is positioned in various ways—supine, sitting, and bending (Figs. 9.5A to C). When the optimum site has been determined, the skin is tattooed with a 27-gauge sterile needle and India ink so that, when the abdomen is opened and the anatomic relationships are distorted, the chosen site will not be mistaken.

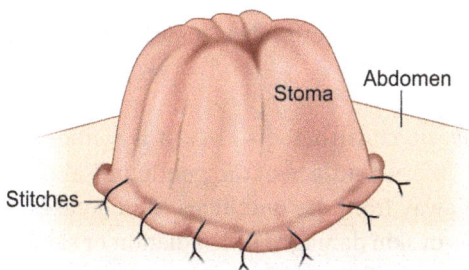

**Fig. 9.1:** Stoma showing stiches attaching bowel to the abdomen

**Flowchart 9.1:** Possible choices of pouching system when the Abdomen is "Firm"

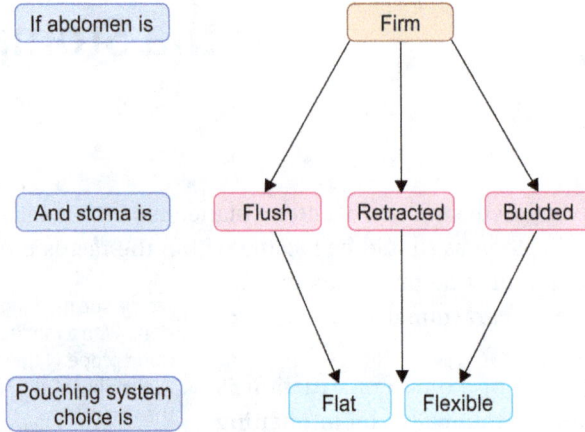

| If abdomen is | Firm |
| And stoma is | Flush / Retracted / Budded |
| Pouching system choice is | Flat / Flexible |

*Source*: Cataldo PA, Meckaigan JM. Intestinal Stomas—Principles, Techniques and Management, 2nd edn, revised and expanded. Stoma Therapy-Ian C Lavery, Paul Erwin-Toth; p. 72.

**Flowchart 9.2:** Possible choices of pouching system when the abdomen is "Soft"

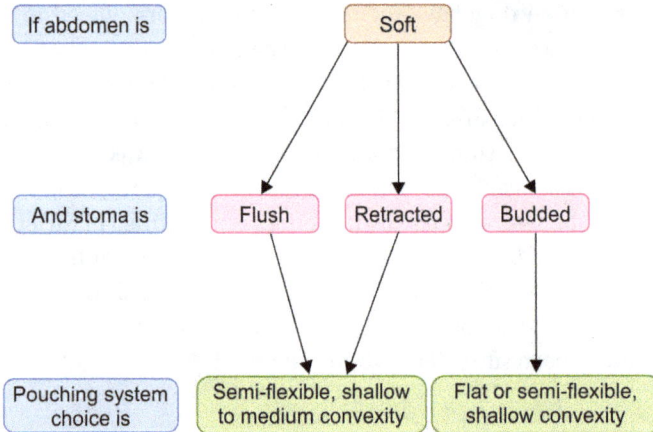

| If abdomen is | Soft |
| And stoma is | Flush / Retracted / Budded |
| Pouching system choice is | Semi-flexible, shallow to medium convexity / Flat or semi-flexible, shallow convexity |

*Source*: Cataldo PA, Meckaigan JM. Intestinal Stomas—Principles, Techniques and Management, 2nd edn, revised and expanded; Stoma Therapy-Ian C Lavery, Paul Erwin-Toth; p. 72.

The stoma must be constructed so that it is visible to the patient (i.e. not located on the inferior surface of the pendulous abdomen). The stoma should be located away from the umbilicus, skin creases, scars, and bony prominences. Areas of skin damaged by irradiation or skin grafts also should be avoided. In the immediate postoperative period, a pectin skin barrier is used for end stomas. A karaya washer is used for loop stomas because, when

**Flowchart 9.3:** Possible choices of Pouching system when the abdomen is "Very soft"

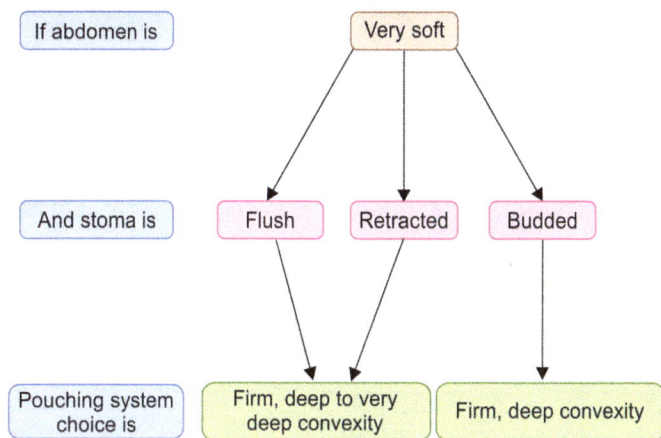

*Source*: Peter A Cataldo, John M Meckaigan. Intestinal Stomas—Principles, Techniques and Management, 2nd edn, revised and expanded; Stoma Therapy-Ian C Lavery, Paul Erwin-Toth; p. 72.

the karaya reaches body temperature, it molds itself over the rod and creates a seal. A temporary ostomy pouch is used until the rod has been removed. When the rod is removed, the patient is fitted with an ostomy management system and given instructions on care of the stoma and the equipment. The patient must be competent and comfortable with care of the stoma before hospital discharge; because deficiencies in care can have serious psychological and physical consequences for the patient. Follow-up in the clinic usually takes place 1 month after discharge, so that the situation can be assessed and the stoma can be remeasured as postoperative edema resolves. If necessary, self-care instruction can be continued by a home care ET nurse. Since construction of a stoma creates an abnormal anatomical situation, complications may occur. However, such complications can be minimized through the surgeon's understanding of physiology and correct construction of the stoma.

## ■ WHERE WILL THE STOMA BE PLACED?

The stoma will be placed on the right or left side of the abdomen. It will be positioned "proximal to" or "above" the area of disease or injury, to enable you to excrete body waste without further pain or infection (Figs. 9.2A and B and 9.3).

Your colostomy may be located in the sigmoid, descending, transverse or ascending colon.

- *Sigmoid colostomy*: For disease or injury to the anus or rectum. Output is usually solid, occurring once or twice a day.

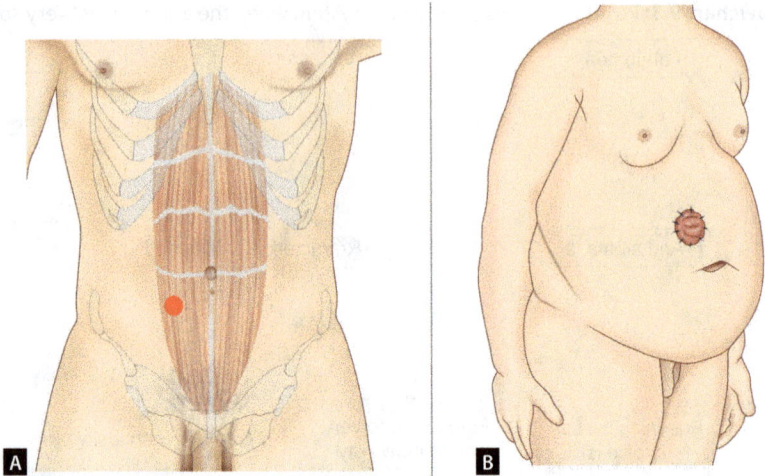

**Figs. 9.2A and B:** (A) The optimum site for an ileostomy is the apex of the subumbilical fat roll through the rectus muscle; (B) In patients with a pendulous abdomen, the stoma needs to be located in the upper abdomen so that it can be seen by the patient. It also needs to be placed in an area of skin that is flat
*Source*: Cataldo PA, Meckaigan JM. Intestinal Stomas—Principles, Techniques and Management; Second edition, revised and expanded; Stoma Therapy-Ian C Lavery, Paul Erwin-Toth; p. 66.

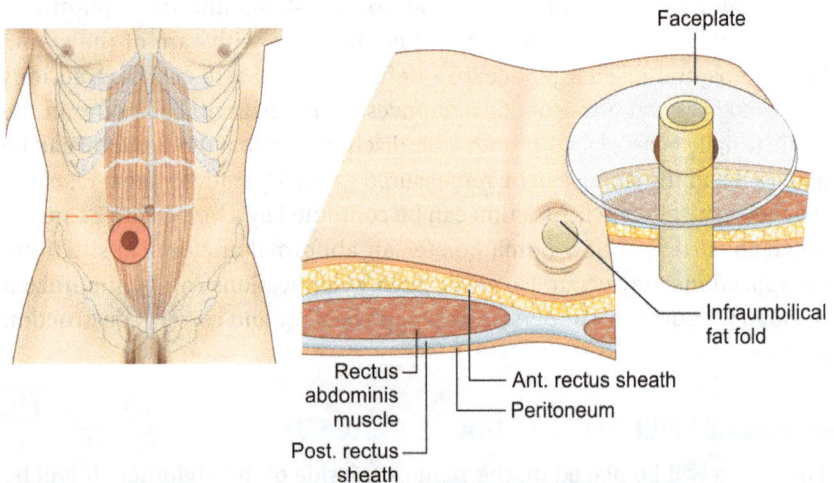

**Fig. 9.3:** Selection of site to bring the stoma through rectus

- *Descending colostomy:* For disease or injury to the sigmoid colon. Output usually solid, occurring once or twice a day.
- *Left or right transverse colostomy*: For disease or trauma in the descending or left transverse colon. Output is usually soft, pasty and may occur 2–4 times a day.

- *Ascending colostomy*: For disease in the transverse or ascending colon. Output is liquid occurring 4–6 times a day.

## ■ STOMA SITE SELECTION (TABLE 9.1 AND FIG. 9.4)

Stoma site selection and marking should be done for all patients scheduled for Ostomy surgery by an experienced, educated, competent clinician. This should be considered even if there is only a possibility for stoma creation. For a pouch to fit

> Better to create an ugly stoma in a good location than a pretty stoma in an ugly location
> *–Peter Cataldo*

comfortably and securely, it is important to have an adequate, intact skin surface. Proper placement helps prevent skin and stoma complications, pouching problems, and pain and clothing concerns. The optimal site enhances the likelihood of independence in stoma care and resumption of normal activities. The preoperative visit also provides an opportunity for education for patient and family.

**Table 9.1:** Do's and Dont's of Stoma site selection

| Ideal stoma characteristics | Sites to avoid | Other considerations |
|---|---|---|
| • Red<br>• Round<br>• Raised (about 1" protrusion)<br>• Lumen at center of stoma<br>• Smooth skin surface | • Scars/wrinkles<br>• Skin folds/creases<br>• Bony prominence<br>• Under pendulous breasts<br>• Suture lines<br>• Umbilicus<br>• Belt/waistline<br>• Hernia<br>• Mobile abdominal tissue<br>• Radiation sites | • Type of ostomy<br>• Occupation<br>• Impairments (e.g. visual, physical)<br>• Sports/activity level<br>• Prosthetic equipment<br>• Preference (surgeon, patient)<br>• Posture<br>• Contractures<br>• Diagnosis<br>• Age |

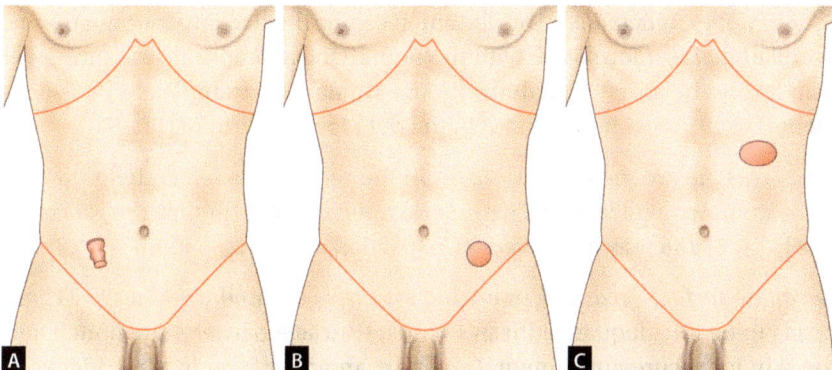

**Figs. 9.4A to C:** Stoma sites for (A) Ileostomy;
(B) Sigmoid colostomy; (C) Transverse colostomy

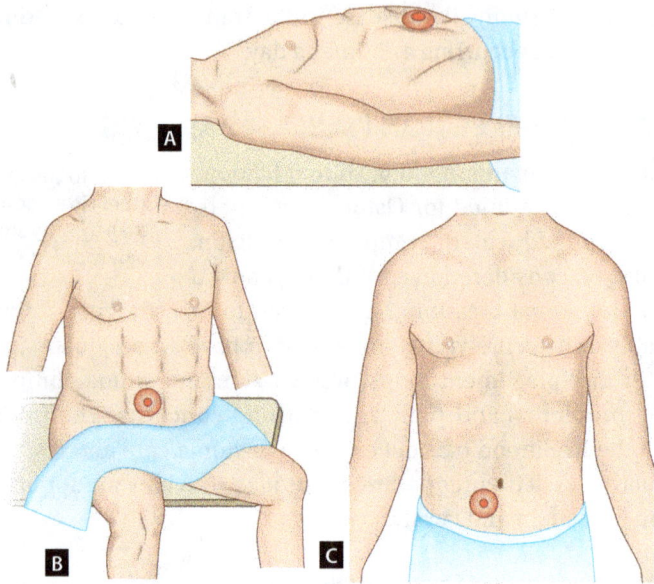

**Figs. 9.5A to C:** Stoma in (A) Lying; (B) Sitting; (C) Standing position

## Desirable Stoma Locations (Fig. 9.7)

• Ileostomy or urostomy (e.g., ileal conduit)
• Sigmoid/descending colostomy
• Transverse colostomy

## Positions

Evaluate potential site in lying, sitting, bending and standing positions.

To select the correct site for the stoma, the following assessments should be made preoperatively:

*Type of stoma anticipated*: The abdomen can be divided into four quadrants. Correlating this information with the underlying anatomical structures, will help locate the correct quadrant for the stoma. For example, an ileostomy (ileum) would usually be located in the right lower quadrant (Fig. 9.6).

*The rectus muscle sheath*: Placement in the rectus muscle can help prevent some stomal complications. This muscle runs vertically through the abdomen (*see* Fig. 9.3) and may be located by inspection and/or palpation.

*Adequate surface area*: The pouching system is secured by adhesive. There needs to be an adequate adhesive contact surface between the pouch and the skin for secure attachment. Generally an area of two to three inches of flat surface is preferred but not always possible. On a child, a smaller area

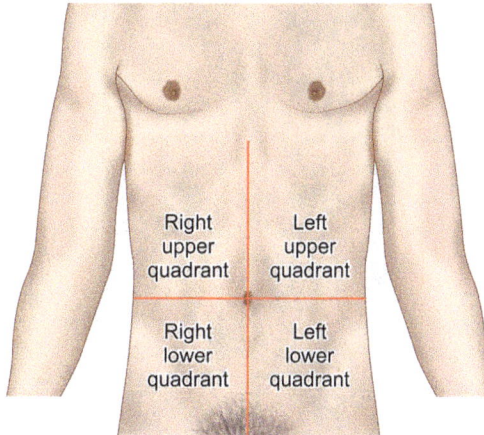

Fig. 9.6: Four quadrants of abdomen

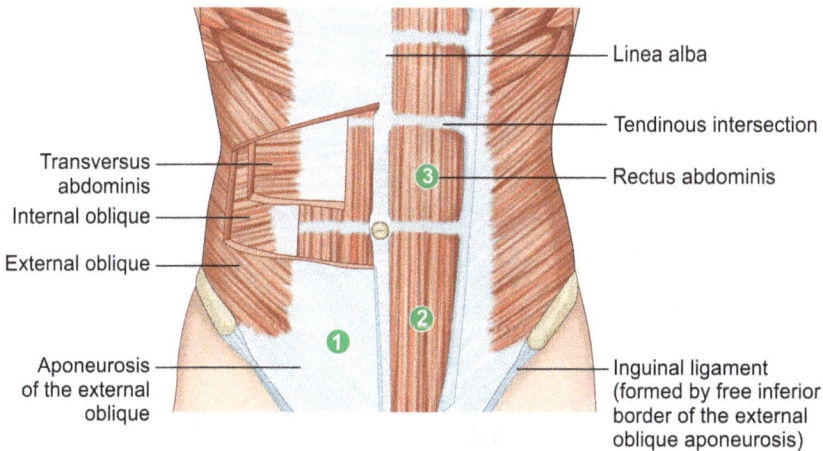

Fig. 9.7: Desirable stoma locations. 1. Ileostomy or urostomy;
2. Sigmoid or descending colostomy; 3. Transverse colostomy

is needed and dependent on body size. A stoma siting disc can be used to evaluate adequate skin surface area preoperatively.

*Easily seen*: It is difficult for a person to be independent in their care if they cannot see their stoma. Select a site visible to the patient and if possible, below the belt line to conceal the pouch. For many people, the best location is in the lower quadrant on the apex of the skin surface. If the patient is extremely obese, location can be placed in the upper quadrant.

*Smooth skin surface*: Locating the stoma in an area where the skin is flat is important. The prospective stoma site should be located away from skin

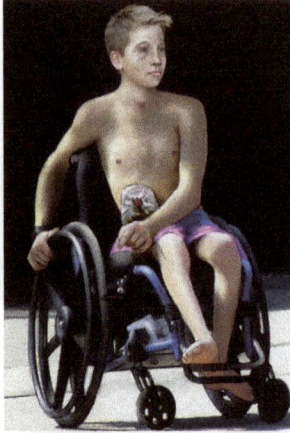

**Fig. 9.8:** Stoma in a physically challenged person

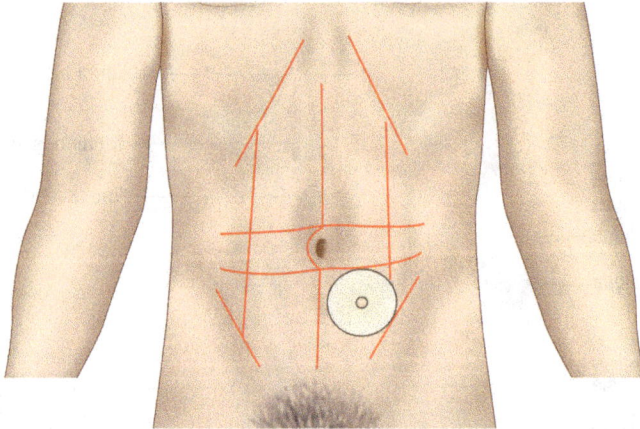

**Fig. 9.9:** Marking of stoma site

folds, bony prominence, scars, the umbilicus, incision lines and the belt line. Any of these can interfere with a secure pouch seal. The abdomen should be observed in various positions.

*Miscellaneous criteria*: In addition there may be other factors that could impact where the stoma would ideally be located. Example: in case of person using a wheelchair, a walker or a brace or who needs more than one stoma. Fecal and urinary stomas should be marked on different horizontal planes/ lines (Fig. 9.8).

*Marking the site*: After the site is selected, it needs to be marked. The technique used for marking the site varies and may be based on hospital protocols (Fig. 9.9). The site location should be documented and communicated to the surgeon so that the intent of the mark is understood in the operating room. An indelible marker or skin dye may be used to identify the site but must be visible after the surgical scrub. In some cases, two choices may be made with the first labeled as #1. Preoperative site markings are a guide. Final selection is done by the surgeon during the operative procedure.

## BIBLIOGRAPHY

1. Carlstedt A, Tasth S, Hulten W, et al. Long-term ileostomy complications in patients with ulcerative colitis and Crohn's disease. Int J Colorectal Dis. 1987;2:22-25.
2. Cataldo PA, Meckaigan JM. Intestinal Stomas—Principles, Techniques and Management, 2nd edn, revised and expanded; Stoma Therapy-Ian C Lavery, Paul Erwin-Toth; p. 72.
3. Goligher JC. Surgery of the Anus, Rectum and Colon, 5th edn. London: Bailliere Tindall. 1984:703-4, 891-4.
4. Horgan K, Hughes LE. Para-ileostomy hernia: failure of a local repair technique. Br J Surg. 1986;73:439-40.
5. Ostomy care tips-Stoma site selection: Hollister education.
6. Prian GW, Sawyer RB, Sawyer, KC. Repair of peristomal colostomy hernias. Am J Surg. 1975;130:694-6.

# Pediatric Stoma Care

Stoma care for adults is now readily available in many countries. But there is a dearth of pediatric nurses working in the stoma care field. The incidence of stoma requirement in children is far less as compared to adult population and it is extremely traumatic time for a family when they come to know that their child require Ostomy surgery. But then they realize over a period of time that this may be the only option for the child to survive.

Although there is high acceptance of Stomas within the adult community (Fig. 10.1), there is a poor acceptance in teenagers who are concerned with their peer acceptance and fragile body images at this age. It is a huge challenge for the family to treat their child who is having a stoma. They have to hone the skills in handling their child's stoma along with the pediatric conditions prevailing with their child.

One has to accept that there are purely physical differences between stomas and their care between adults and children, especially the tiny appliances which are difficult to source and care. The skin of children is very fine and less resilient so that the stoma care must be meticulous. The mother should know to empty the bag before nap time, bedtime or going out door.

Infants have different abdominal dimensions and musculature. The abdominal wall is very thin and the muscles give poor support for the stomas making prolapse much more common.

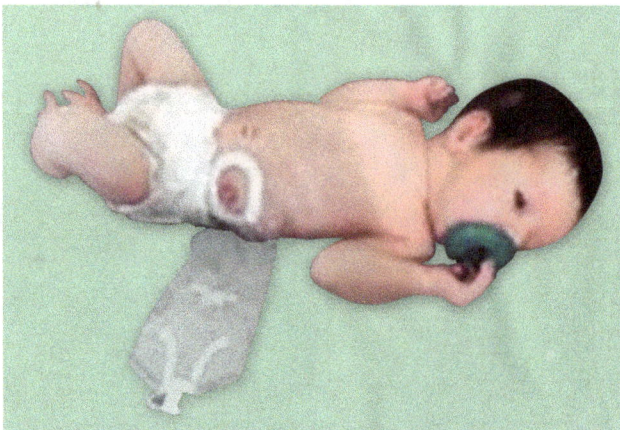

**Fig. 10.1:** Baby with a colostomy bag

It is difficult to site the stoma as ideally as an adult with regard to the umbilicus and pelvic bones. One should know that in children the stoma must be placed within the operative wound as opposed to a separate incision due to lack of space. Hence the pediatric stomas are much more difficult to look after, because all care is done by the child's carers and the stomas are more difficult to fit and keep on.

In children the stoma could be temporary or permanent. In temporary stoma the gut has a period of rest and recovery. In permanent stoma the child has to carry the stoma throughout its life.

## ■ CONDITIONS THAT NECESSITATE A STOMA

### Imperforate Anus

When there is no exit for the bowel and its contents (Fig. 10.2).

### Hirschsprung's Disease

This is a disease which affects the large intestine (colon) thereby causing difficulties in passing stool. This condition is present since birth as a result of absence of nerve cells in the muscular coat of the colon (Fig. 10.3).

### Inflammatory Bowel Disease (Fig. 10.4)

It comprises a group of intestinal disorders where there is chronic inflammation of the alimentary canal. This commonly includes Crohn's disease and ulcerative colitis.

### Neonatal Necrotising Enterocolitis

This disease occurs in premature babies and formula –fed infants where in there is a considerable damage to the intestinal tract from mucosa to full thickness of the bowel. Hence the babies require stoma to lead a normal life.

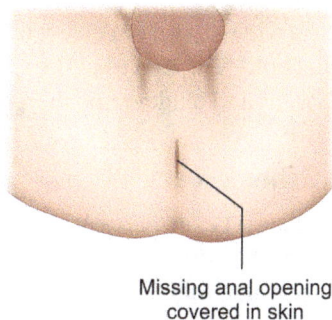

Missing anal opening
covered in skin

**Fig. 10.2:** Imperforate anus

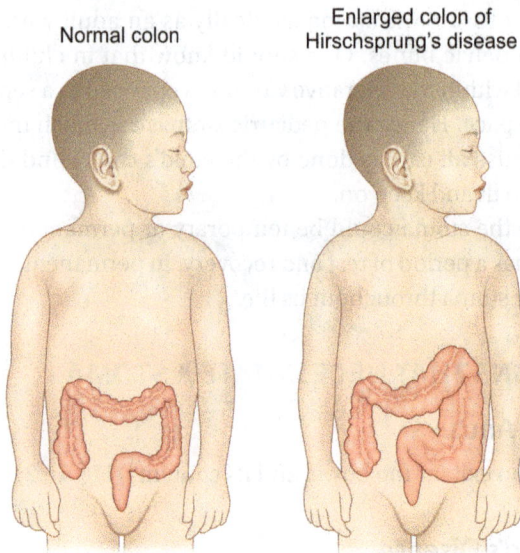

Normal colon

Enlarged colon of Hirschsprung's disease

**Fig. 10.3:** Hirschsprung's disease

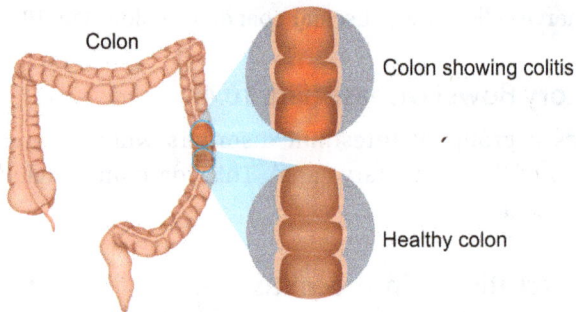

Colon

Colon showing colitis

Healthy colon

**Fig. 10.4:** Ulcerative colitis

## Spina Bifida (Fig. 10.5)

This is a congenital disease where there is a defect in the formation of bones of the spine and the spinal cord. The nerves of the spinal cord fail to control the muscles of the legs, bowels and bladder and therefore a stoma is required.

## Accident Injury and Other Causes

Injuries to the bladder and bowel which are caused by accidents may end up causing damage to these organs impairing the passage of stool and urine as well as their control. To overcome this stoma is created for collection of stool and urine.

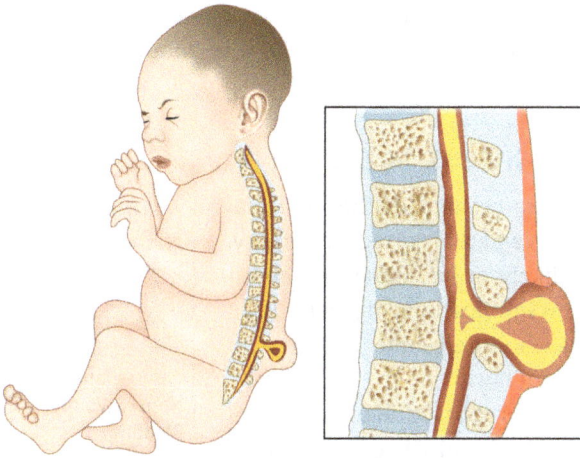

**Fig. 10.5:** Spinabifida

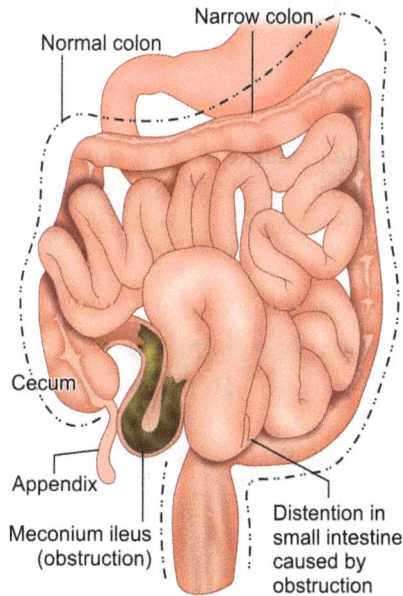

**Fig. 10.6:** Meconium ileus

## Meconium Ileus

Cystic fibrosis is a genetically determined disease which affects Intestinal, Bronchial, Salivary and Sweat glands and the Pancreas. Sometimes they present with intestinal obstruction requiring stoma surgery (Fig. 10.6).

To relieve the obstruction a temporary loop Ileostomy will be created and enable washouts to be done via the stoma. The stoma is normally closed once the baby is thriving.

## SPECIFIC ASPECTS OF STOMA CARE

Most stomas are created in the neonatal period – often as a part of corrective surgery. Families are likely to be concerned about the nature and implications of their child's condition as a whole and come to terms with the situation generally.

Most principles of practical management of stomal appliances and skin care described in the adults are also applicable when considered for children. But in the pediatric age group the stoma care differs from Infants up to Adolescence.

> **Points to note during post-operative period**
> Bleeding, Fever, Redness swelling and discharge from the wound, color of stoma, Signs of dehydration, Watery stool, no gas or effluent from the stoma, Nausea, Vomiting, Cramping or Bloating.
> These conditions warrant vigilance and needs to be attended immediately

### Infants

Generally 1 piece flexible pediatric or mini stoma bags are more suitable for the size and shape of babies. Since babies skin dry easily, hence alcohol based agents such as adhesive removers and skin protective wipes should not be used (Fig. 10.7).

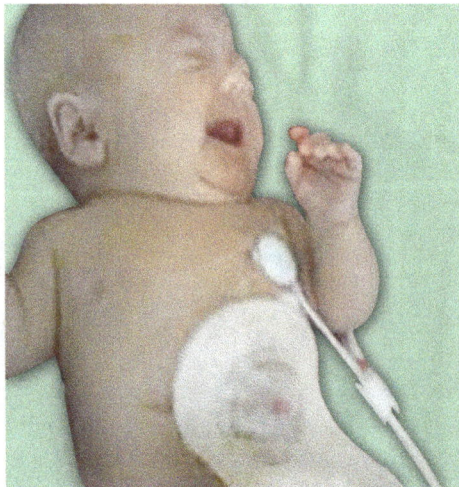

**Fig. 10.7:** Infant with stoma bag

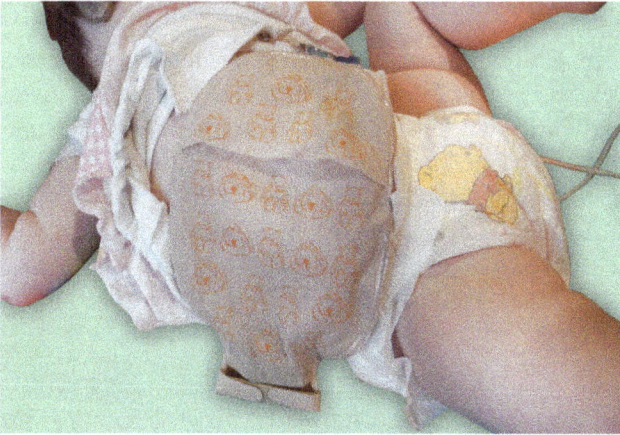

**Fig. 10.8:** Children's stoma bag

Parents should be encouraged to aid bonding and appropriate care and love to come to term with their baby's condition. As the children grow the stomal output increases and the appliances will need regular reviewing.

## 6 Months to 2 Years

Children of this age always prefer familiar faces in family and care givers to help them feel secured. Positive messages about the stoma and equipment should be conveyed during appliance changes (Fig. 10.8).

## Age 2–5 Years

Children of this age are curious about their own and their friend's bodies and may ask why they function differently. Parents can be encouraged to offer simple explanations bearing in mind that a child's attention span is about 10–15 minutes in 3 years and increases correspondingly at the age of 5.

The children should be taught to promote self-care as they prepare for nursery and school attendance. The school personnel should be informed about child's condition so that they can call on the expertise of the patient and stoma nurse when required.

## Age 6–12 years

Many children of this age group will have had their stoma for some time. Here, parents and children need help to make the transition from parents doing the stoma care to the child, gaining ability to manage their own care.

## Adolescence

An adolescent with stoma wants himself to be identical with his peer group with a developing sense of themselves physically, sexually and emotionally. They wish to be accepted, looking and behaving like their friends and maintain equally well in their studies and friendships retaining their self-esteem.

Though they are wise enough to manage their stoma independently their only concern at this stage is to tell their friends about their condition, fit their stoma and its management discretely into sports and social activities and to feel confident of themselves.

**Points to remember**
- After surgery your child will pass stool/urine through the stoma instead and will not be able to control when these occur. To help with this a pouch is worn to collect the waste.
- It is common for the stoma and the area around it to be slightly swollen for around 6-8 weeks after surgery after which the swelling will subside.
- Stomas have no nerve endings and therefore no feeling. So it will not hurt when touched.
- Depending on the type of stoma, the output will be different.
- The stoma may grow with your child especially if it is permanent. It is important therefore to re-measure the stoma from time to time to ensure that the pouch still fits correctly
- At times when your child is crying you may notice a color change in the color of the stoma. However, the normal colour will return when the crying stops

http://www.eakincohesiveseals.com/what-to-expect-when-your-child-needs-a-stoma

## ■ BIBLIOGRAPHY

1. Caring for your child with an ostomy: Hollister.
2. Colostomy Care in Paediatric Patients. International Journal of Science and Research. (IJSR) ISSN (Online): 2319-7064 Index Copernicus Value (2013): 6.14 | Impact Factor (2014): 5.611.
3. Gastrointestinal Stomas in Children—CHAPTER 72 Osarumwense David Osifo Johanna R. Askegard-Giesmann Benedict C. Nwomeh
4. http://www.eakincohesiveseals.com/what-to-expect-when-your-child-needs-a-stoma
5. Stomas of small and large intestine in children. http://emedicine.medscape.com/article/939455-overview.

# Pouching System Procedures

## ■ INTRODUCTION

General issues that must be considered in establishing pouching system procedures include the following: organizational matters, timing of pouch change, frequency of pouch change, and sizing of the pouch or barrier opening.

> Choice of the pouch depends on the stoma and it is better to throw the choice of pouch to patients as well.

## ■ TYPES OF POUCHING SYSTEMS (FIGS. 11.1, 11.2A AND B)

Pouching systems may include a one-piece or two-piece system. Both kinds include a skin barrier/wafer ("faceplate" in older terminology) and a collection pouch.

The pouch (one-piece or two-piece) attaches to the abdomen by the skin barrier and is fitted over and around the stoma to collect the diverted output, either stool or urine.

The barrier/wafer is designed to protect the skin from the stoma output and to be as neutral to the skin as possible.

### Colostomy and Ileostomy Pouches

Can be either open-ended, requiring a closing device (traditionally a clamp or tail clip); or closed and sealed at the bottom. Open-ended pouches are called drainable and are left attached to the body while emptying. Closed end pouches are most commonly used by colostomates who can irrigate or by patients who have regular elimination patterns. Closed end pouches are usually discarded after one use.

> Preoperative mock session of handling fluid filled bag to be carried out with patients' to prepare them mentally for the postoperative phase.

### Organization of Materials (Fig. 11.3)

It is helpful to organize all the products required for the pouch changing procedure in one area and to assemble all necessary supplies before the procedure is begun. Necessary supplies include a plastic trash bag (for disposing of soiled items), a wet washcloth or disposable wipes, the pouch itself, and any products for skin protection (e.g., skin barrier powder, sealants,

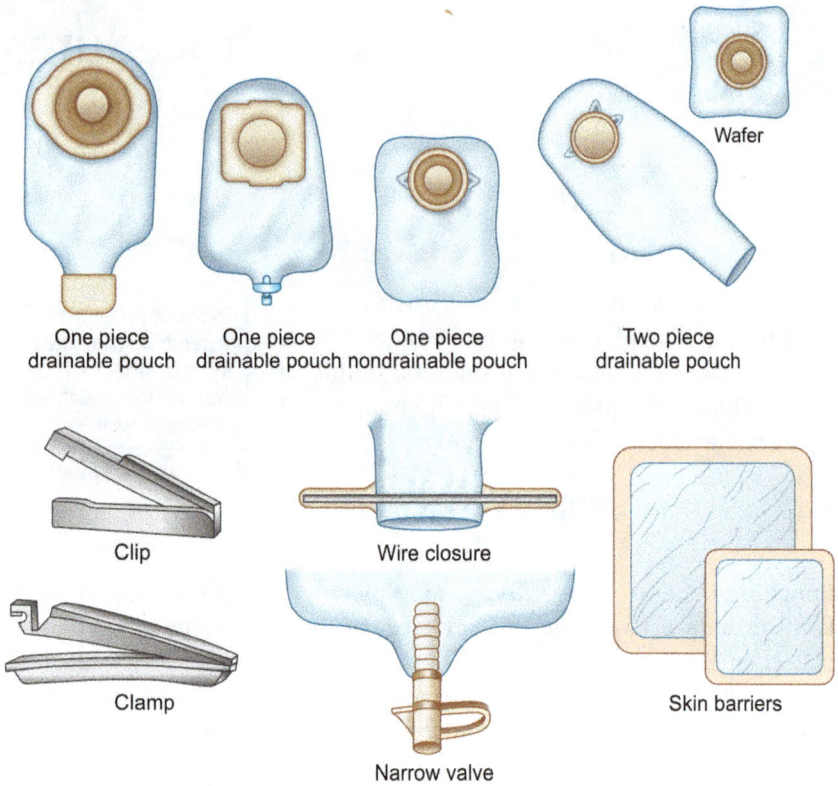

One piece
drainable pouch

One piece
drainable pouch

One piece
nondrainable pouch

Two piece
drainable pouch

Wafer

Clip

Clamp

Wire closure

Narrow valve

Skin barriers

**Fig. 11.1:** Ostomy pouches and accessories

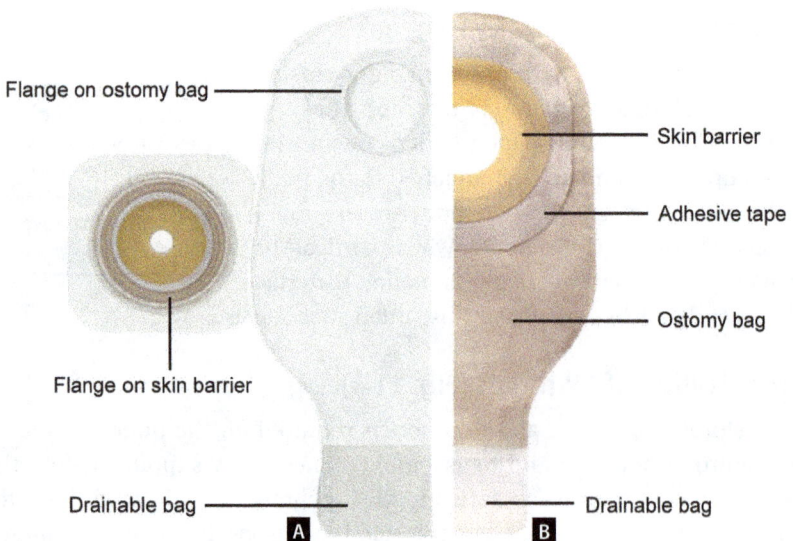

Flange on ostomy bag

Flange on skin barrier

Skin barrier

Adhesive tape

Ostomy bag

Drainable bag

Drainable bag

A

B

**Figs. 11.2A and B:** (A) Two-piece ostomy bag; (B) One-piece ostomy bag

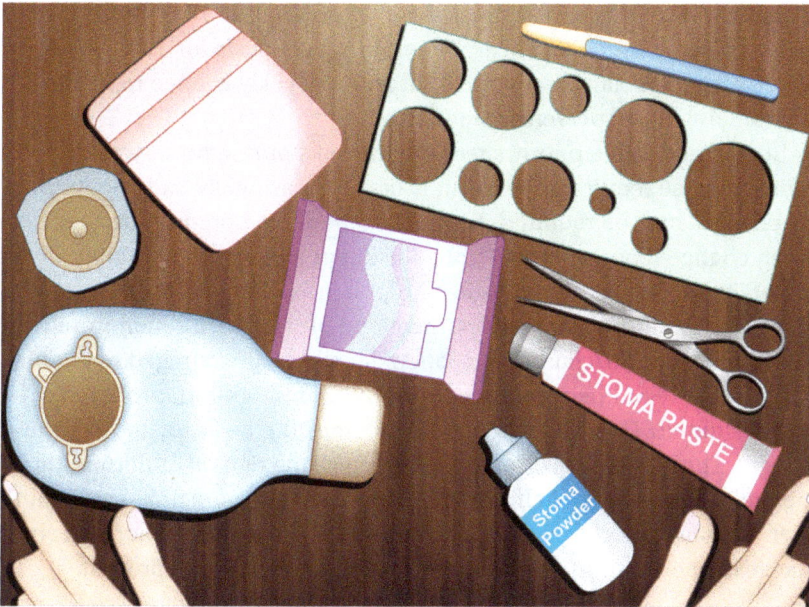

**Fig. 11.3:** Organization of materials

or paste). When a cut-to-fit pouch is used, a measuring guide or pattern, pencil, and scissors are also needed. If hair is present in the peristomal area, an electric or disposable razor may be required. When a pouch is to be applied to a urinary stoma or a high-output fecal stoma, it is advisable to have an ample supply of absorbent materials, such as soft paper towels, nonsterile gauze, tampons, or dental wicks.

## Timing of Pouch Change

Optimally, the pouch is changed when the stoma is not highly active. A fecal stoma is usually most active within 2, hr of a meal. For a urinary stoma, the best time for a pouch change is usually early in the morning, before fluid consumption. Each patient learns his or her own best time for pouch changes.

## Frequency of Pouch Change

There is no "correct" frequency for pouch changes. The goal is to establish a routine schedule that prevents leakage and provides the individual with control. According to recent global guidelines it is recommended to change the pouch with the

Humid and hot climate would force the patient to change the pouch earlier as compared to those in cooler places.

Conditions that may demand a change of pouch:
1. Itching sensation
2. Burning sensation around the base plate
3. When looking forward for long hours of journey
4. When the pouch is not inflated, hinting a leak

frequency of 3–5 days based on the skin condition. With more durable products, some individuals can maintain secure seals for 10 days or even longer. Most clinicians recommend at least a weekly change to inspect the peristomal skin and prevent irritation.

In contrast, with a poorly sited or retracted stoma, a twice-weekly pouch change may be required to prevent leakage; occasionally daily or alternate-day changes may be required. Establishment of the optimum frequency for pouch change requires individual adjustment and experimentation. In the immediate postoperative period, the pouch is changed more frequently than usual to permit stoma assessment and provide instruction in self-care procedures. After discharge, the patient should be encouraged to gradually extend the interval between pouch changes until optimum frequency can be determined. This frequency then becomes the basis for routine pouch changes. The patient is also taught to recognize the signs of undermining and impending leakage (i.e., itching or burning of the peristomal skin, odor noted when the pouch is closed, or visible "meltdown" of the skin barrier) and to change the pouch promptly whenever any of these signs are present.

## Sizing of Pouch or Barrier Opening (Figs. 11.4 and 11.5)

Most manufacturers of ostomy supplies include disposable stoma-measuring guides in each box of pouches. These guides are used to determine the size of a round stoma. An opening that clears the stoma and minimizes exposure of the peristomal skin should be selected. For irregularly shaped stomas, it is necessary to make a pattern that can be used to size the barrier or pouch opening. One simple way to make a pattern is to use a transparent piece of

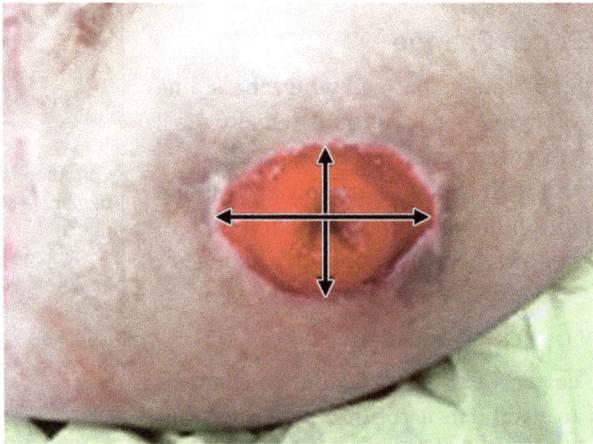

**Fig. 11.4:** How to determine the stoma size

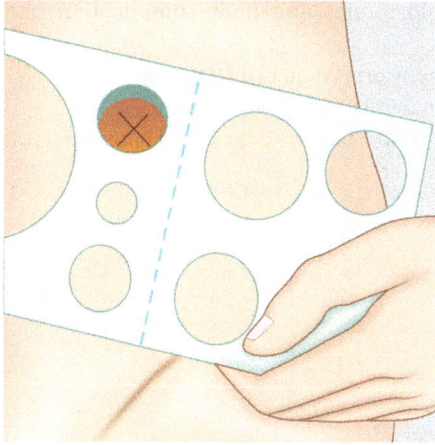

**Fig. 11.5:** Using a gauge

plastic and a felt-tipped marker to trace the contours of the stoma. The pattern is then cut out and altered as necessary until a good fit has been obtained. The pattern should be labeled with arrows indicating "head" and "foot" and "pouch side" and "skin side."

When a barrier is added to an adhesive pouch, the barrier is sized to fit closely around the stoma without impinging on the bowel mucosa; the pouch is sized to clear the stoma by at least 1/8 inch. This method prevents the rigid pouch opening from causing damage to the stoma; in addition, it prevents tunneling of the effluent between the barrier and the pouch. Because edema decreases during the first 6–8 weeks after surgery, the size of the stoma decreases and the opening of the ostomy device must be resized at each pouch change during this period. Once shrinkage is complete, further resizing is not necessary unless the stoma changes. The condition of a patient who is not able to measure the stoma or who has an irregularly shaped stoma must be followed closely during the first 6–8 weeks after surgery, either by a home care nurse or through follow-up at an outpatient clinic.

## ■ BIBLIOGRAPHY

1. Beck DE, Fazio VW, Grundfest-Broniatowski S. Surgical management of bleeding stomal varices. Dis Colon Rectum. 1988;31:343-6.
2. Cataldo PA, Meckaigan JM. Intestinal Stomas—Principles, Techniques and Management; second edition, revised and expanded; Stoma Therapy-Ian C Lavery, Paul Erwin-Toth; pp. 69, 70.
3. Goligher JC. Surgery of the Anus, Rectum and Colon, 5th edn. London: Bailliere Tindall. 1984:7034, 891-4.

4. Green EW. Colostomies and their complication. Surg Gynecol Obstet. 1966;1:1230-2.
5. http://www.ostomy.org/What_is_an_Ostomy.html
6. http://www.spinabifidainfo.nl/ostomy.html
7. Prian GW, Sawyer RB, Sawyer, KC. Repair of peristomal colostomy hernias. Am J Surg. 1975;130:694-6.

# Application of Stoma Products

Stoma products are divided into:

a. One–piece system
b. Two–piece system

## ■ APPLICATION OF ONE-PIECE FECAL POUCH

### One-Piece Systems

Consist of a skin barrier/wafer and pouch joined together as a single unit. Provide greater simplicity than two-piece systems but require changing the entire unit, including skin barrier, when the pouch is changed.

1. Gather all supplies.
2. Gently remove soiled pouch by pushing down on skin while lifting up on pouch. Discard soiled pouch in odor proof plastic bag. Save tail closure (Figs. 12.1 to 12.3).
3. Clean stoma and peristomal skin with water; pat dry. If indicated, shave or clip peristomal hair (Fig. 12.4).
4. Use stoma-measuring guide or established pattern to determine size of stoma. *Pre-sized pouch*: Check to be sure pouch opening is correct size. Order new supplies if indicated (Fig. 12.5).
5. *Cut-to-fit pouch*: Trace correctly sized pattern onto back of barrier or pouch surface and cut stomal opening to match pattern. Once stomal shrinkage is complete, this step may be omitted and preparation of the clean pouch may be completed before the soiled pouch is removed.

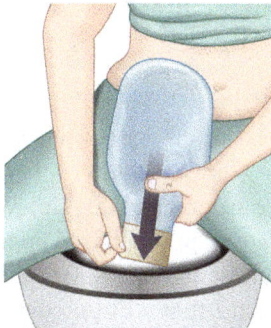

**Fig. 12.1:** Emptying the stool from the pouch in the toilet

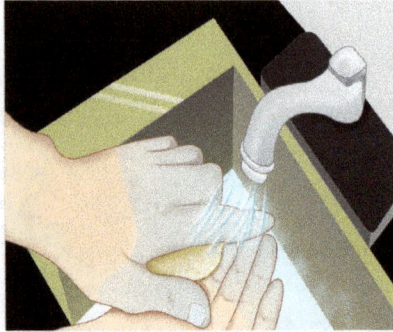

**Fig. 12.2:** Washing hands with soap and water or with antibacterial sanitizer to maintain proper hygiene

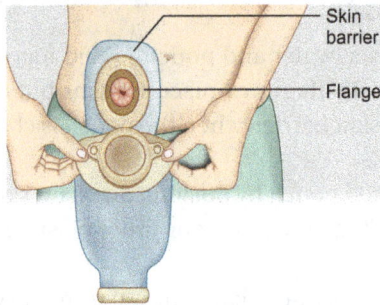

**Fig. 12.3:** Removing the pouch after emptying

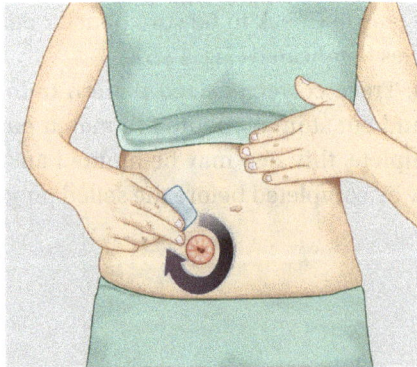

**Fig. 12.4:** Cleaning the skin surrounding the stoma

6. Apply skin barrier paste around stoma. (Tip: wet finger to facilitate paste application.) An alternative approach is to apply skin barrier paste to the aperture in the prepared pouch or barrier. Allow paste to dry. Optional: Apply skin sealant to skin that will be covered by tape. Allow to dry (Fig. 12.6).

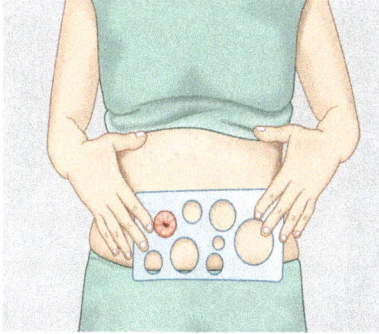

**Fig. 12.5:** Measuring the size of the stoma using stoma measuring guide

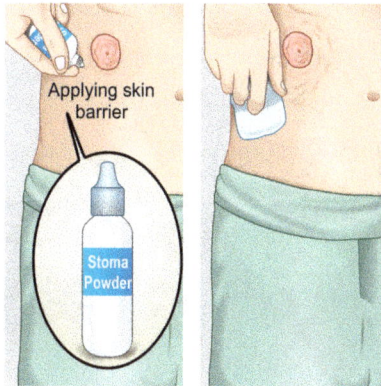

**Fig. 12.6:** Applying skin barrier

7. Remove paper backing from pouch or barrier to expose adhesive surface; center pouch opening over stoma and press into place. Attach closure. Optional: Apply tape strips to ' "picture frame" the pouch-skin junction (Figs. 12.7 and 12.8).

## Pouch System Options for Urinary Stoma

In applying a pouch to a urinary stoma, two approaches can be taken:
1. A pouch with an attached skin barrier can be used (the skin barrier is sized to fit snugly around the stoma) or
2. An adhesive-only system with an anti-reflux valve can be used. In the latter approach, the pouch opening is sized to adhere to a flat abdominal surface, even if cutting of the pouch opening wide and exposure of the skin are required. Both approaches are valid because the intent of each is to protect the skin from pooled urine. Skin barriers are not always

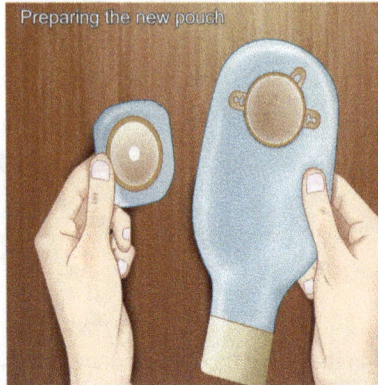

**Fig. 12.7:** Preparing the new pouch

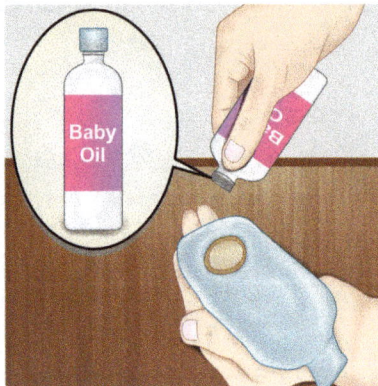

**Fig. 12.8:** Baby oil keeps the stool from sticking to the bag

required, but their use may increase the wearing time of the pouching system. Pouches with barriers are sized to fit closely around the stoma because the barriers are moldable and usually can adapt to peristomal contours.

3. If the stoma is protruding (budded) and the pouch is equipped with an anti-reflux valve, any barrier that adheres well to the peristomal skin is appropriate.

For example, karaya and pectin barriers are known to break down as a result of exposure to urine; however, they may be effective with a budded stoma if the pouch is equipped with an anti-reflux valve (because the urine projects into the pouch and backflow is limited by the anti-reflux valve). With a flush or skin-level stoma, however, it is important to select a barrier that is resistant to breakdown by urine. Urine from a flush stoma constantly washes over the barrier, and a barrier that is not resistant to urine quickly deteriorates

**Table 12.1:** Showing pouch selection criteria and options

| *Pouching selection* | *Pouching options* |
|---|---|
| • Type of stoma | • Drainable vs Urostomy vs Closed |
| • Abdominal contours | • One vs two piece |
| • Stoma characteristics | • Pre-cut vs cut to fit |
| • Patient/caregiver abilities | • Accessories |
| • Preference | • Daily change |

(Table 12.1). When a pouch with a barrier is being changed, the barrier and the peristomal skin are assessed to ascertain that the barrier is not absorbing the urine and causing peristomal maceration. Some patients with urinary stomas obtain longer pouch seals and improved skin protection by using adhesive-only pouching systems with a "hydrophobic" barrier. In the application of an adhesive-only pouch with an anti-reflux valve, the goal is to obtain a good seal between the pouch and the peristomal skin in order to prevent pooling of urine. Adhesive surfaces cannot adapt to changing peristomal contours. If they are applied over irregular contours and deep creases, they may become partially detached and allow pooling. The pouch opening should be sized to permit adherence to a flat abdominal pouching surface. It must be emphasized that this approach requires the use of a pouch with an anti-reflux valve; backflow of urine must be prevented because the peristomal skin is exposed. The use of sealants or cements usually is recommended to further protect the skin from maceration.

## Two-Piece Systems

Allow changing pouches, while leaving the barrier/wafer attached to the skin. The wafer/barrier is part of a "flange" unit. The pouches include a closing ring that attaches mechanically to a mating piece on the flange. A common connection mechanism consists of a pressure fit snap ring, similar to that used in Tupperware™.

## Application of One-Piece Urinary Pouch

1. Gather all supplies.
2. Gently remove soiled pouch by pushing down on skin while lifting up on pouch. Discard soiled pouch.
3. Use stoma-measuring guide or establish pattern to determine size of stoma. Pre-sized pouch: Check to be sure,

1. Patients opting for Belt bag should wear it tightly and it is not odor proof
2. If the stoma is not protruding, then Belt bag is not the right choice
3. Skin problems arising due to continuous use of Belt bag may prevent the use of sticky bag.
4. Sizes of the Belt bag are not tailor made for Stoma

pouch opening is correct size. Order new supplies if indicated. Cut-to-fit pouch: Trace correctly sized pattern onto back of pouch and cut stomal opening to match pattern. Once stomal shrinkage is complete, this step may be omitted. If a cut-to-fit pouch is used, pouch may be cut out before soiled pouch is removed.

4. Remove paper backing from pouch, and lay pouch to one side.
5. Clean stoma and peristomal skin with water; pat dry. If indicated, shave or clip peristomal hair. Use wicks against stoma to absorb urine and to keep skin dry for steps 6 and 7.
6. Optional: Apply skin sealant to skin that will be covered by tape. Allow to dry.
7. Remove paper backing from pouch; center pouch opening over stoma and press pouch into place.
8. *Optimal*: Apply tape strips to "picture frame" the pouch-skin junction. Universal precautions must be followed when this procedures is performed. (*Source:* From Erwin-Toth P, Doughty DB. Principles and procedures of stomal management.In: Hampton BG, Bryant RA, eds. Ostomies and Continent Diversions. St Louis: Mosby–Year Book, 1992:59.)

## ■ BIBLIOGRAPHY

1. Basic Ostomy skin care-A guide for Patients and Health care providers-Wound Ostomy and Continence Nurses Society.
   www.wocn.org/?page=BasicOstomySkinCare
2. Cataldo PA, Meckaigan JM. Intestinal Stomas—Principles, Techniques and Management; second edition, revised and expanded; Stoma Therapy-Ian C Lavery, Paul Erwin-Toth.
3. Colostomy care-What you need to know-Drugs.com
   www.drugs.com/cg/colostomy-care.html
4. How to apply (change) a colostomy bag - Ostomy Supplies and Products
   http://www.ostomysoftware.com/OstomyArticles/apply_ostomy_bag.html
5. How to change a colostomy bag:12 steps-wiki how
   jibingso.com/info/0f230ed1bd9c50c85d2fa9909e747cb2.html

# Surgical Principles of Stoma

## ■ INTRODUCTION

The indications of stoma formation are due to various causes. Colorectal cancer is one of the common diseases which need stoma either temporarily or permanently. The other conditions which also need stoma are, inflammatory bowel disease (IBD), diverticular disease, familial adenomatosis polyposis (FAP) and trauma (Table 13.1).

There are two types of stoma; one is temporary in which stoma can be reversed after it serves the purpose. The other is permanent where there is no bowel for anastomosis to the proximal segment and hence the end portion of the bowel has to be fashioned as a permanent stoma.

Stoma after abdomino perineal resection in distal rectal cancer and total procto colectomy with end ileostomy is another example.

## ■ TEMPORARY STOMAS (TABLE 13.2)

Temporary stomas are used to divert the fecal stream from the distal bowel. The following are indications:

- To rest a distal segment of bowel that may be involved in a disease process-such as intestinal fistula or acute Crohn's disease.
- To protect the anastomosis when we predict inadequate blood supply, local sepsis, tension in the anastomosis, elderly patients, during emergency surgery when the patient undergoes pre-operative neoadjuvant chemo-radiation, when there is a distal obstruction.

**Principles of stoma surgery**
- Midline vertical incision
- Adequate blood supply on either side (skin and bowel) without tension
- Avoid pre-existing infection
- Avoid too small hole at fascial level
- No twist of the bowel for Stoma
- Stoma hole at the end of the surgery

**Preoperative counseling**
- Involve ET nurse
- Misconceptions of stoma
- Quality of life
- Knowledge of disease
- Why stoma is required?
- About surgery, stoma looks, function (visual aids)

## ■ METHODS OF STOMA CONSTRUCTION

*The stoma construction can be performed by different methods.*

1. Through laparotomy; 2. Through laparoscopy; and 3. Through a small incision at the site of stoma. (Trephine)

**Table 13.1:** Showing diseases for stoma surgery, indications and types of stoma

| Disease | Presentation | Indication | Stoma type | Intention |
|---|---|---|---|---|
| Colorectal cancer | Perforation<br>Obstruction<br>Rectal cancer | 1. Defunctioning of bowel<br>2. Relief of obstruction<br>3. Low tumor<br>4. Defunctioning of low anastomosis | 1. Loop or end colostomy<br>2. Loop or end colostomy<br>3. End colostomy<br>4. Loop Ileostomy or colostomy | 1. Temporary often permanent<br>2. Temporary<br>3. Permanent<br>4. Temporary |
| Diverticular disease | Perforation<br>Obstruction<br>Elective resection for fistula | 1. Resolution of sepsis; defunctioning of bowel<br>2. Relief of obstruction<br>3. Protection of anastomosis | 1. Colostomy<br>2. Loop or end colostomy<br>3. Loop ileostomy or colostomy | 1. Temporary sometimes permanent<br>2. Temporary sometimes permanent<br>3. Temporary |
| Ulcerative colitis | 1. Acute colitis<br>2. Chronic colitis | 1. Defunctioning of bowel<br>2. Eradication of disease<br>3. Ileo anal pouch procedure | 1. End ileostomy (after subtotal colostomy)<br>2. End ileostomy (after panproctocolectomy)<br>3. Loop ileostomy | 1. Temporary or permanent<br>2. Permanent<br>3. Temporary |
| Crohn's disease | 1. Crohn colitis<br>2. Small bowel disease<br>3. Perianal disease<br>4. Elective resections for septic complications | • Defunctioning of bowel<br>• Defunctioning of bowel after excision<br>• Defunctioning of bowel<br>• Defunctioning of bowel<br>• Excision of disease<br>• Defunctioning of bowel | • Loop or split ileostomy<br>• End ileostomy or colostomy<br>• Loop, end or split ileostomy<br>• Loop or split ileostomy<br>• Ileostomy ( after panproctocolostomy)<br>• Colostomy (after rectal excision)<br>• Loop or divided loop Ileostomy | • Temporary sometimes permanent<br>• Temporary often permanent<br>• Temporary sometimes permanent<br>• Temporary often permanent<br>• Permanent<br>• Temporary |
| Trauma | Colon injury<br>Rectal injury | Defunctioning of bowel<br>Defunctioning of bowel | Loop Ileostomy or colostomy<br>Colostomy | Temporary sometimes permanent<br>Temporary sometimes permanent |
| Functional disorders | Fecal incontinence<br>Sphincter repair | Defunctioning of anus<br>Defunctioning of bowel | End colostomy<br>Loop ileostomy or colostomy | Permanent<br>Temporary |

**Table 13.2:** Indications for fecal diversion

| |
|---|
| **1. Obstruction**<br>Congenital<br>Neoplastic<br>Inflammatory<br>Ischemic |
| **2. Inflammatory disease complications**<br>Perforation<br>Fistula |
| **3. Traumatic**<br>Trauma<br>Iatrogenic |
| **4. Operative planned**<br>Abdomino perineal resection<br>Total proctocolectomy with end ileostomy<br>Protective diversion |
| **5. Miscellaneous**<br>Volvulus<br>Colonic inertia<br>Rectal fistula<br>Incontinence<br>Paraplegia<br>Decubitus ulcers<br>Burns |

The method of performance of stoma will depend upon the access for surgery. For example, during abdominoperineal resection of rectum through laparotomy, the stoma is constructed after completion of the surgery.

The construction of stoma during a laparoscopic surgery is done laparoscopically as a Minimal invasive procedure. Sometimes, colostomy through a Trephine approach, gives relief of obstruction to the large bowel thereby allowing a definitive procedure through laparoscopic or open method after the patient's condition turns stable.

For all types of stoma the patient should ideally be counseled by the stoma nurse and the site of the stoma marked before the operation (Fig. 13.1).

Prior to surgery, it is important to mark the site of stoma so that the surgeon can construct an ideal stoma. One has

**Colostomy**
- Effluent less corrosive to the skin
- Usual formed stool, closed pouch, 3x daily
- Transverse colostomy may need drainable pouch
- Some patients may opt for irrigation
- *Constipation*: Diet, fluids, drugs, age, mechanical e.g. Hernia, stricture, adhesions

*Treatment*: Oral laxatives/microlax enemas/suppositories

*Diarrhea*
- Right sided/transverse stomas
- Chemotherapy/radiotherapy
- Infection – stool sample
- Drugs, diet, stress, malabsorption, disease e.g. Crohn's, cancer, sub acute obstruction
- Treatment - Imodium

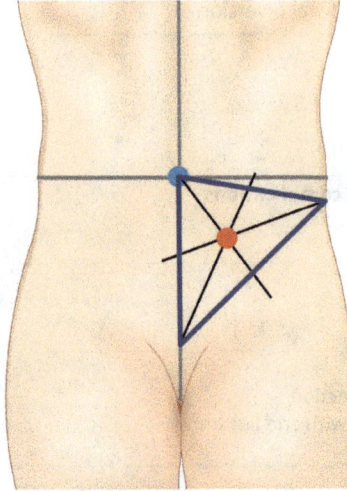

**Fig. 13.1:** Marking of Stoma site before surgery

to remember the rules of marking the stoma site pre-operatively with the patient in sitting, standing and lying position and also to follow all the rules of avoiding improper sites that is mentioned in the previous chapters.

## End Colostomy at Open Surgery

To perform an end colostomy during open surgery, the following steps should be undertaken (Fig. 13.2 and Table 13.2A).

1. After laparotomy the proximal bowel to the area of pathology should be carefully mobilised. For example for a sigmoid colostomy the descending colon, splenic flexure and distal third of the transverse colon should be adequately mobilised based on the middle colic artery.

   Then the pathological area is divided with adequate margin either by stapler or by bowel clamps.

2. After removing the pathological specimen the proximal end of the bowel is brought out as a stoma through the anterior abdominal wall after incising the stoma site, removing a disc of skin and subcutaneous tissue. A cruciate incision given on the anterior rectal sheath and the rectus muscle is split in a longitudinal direction without injuring the muscle.

   Incision is given over the peritoneum and the proximal end of the bowel is brought out through Babkock forceps through the stomal opening located outside.

   One has to be very cautious that the bowel should not be twisted while performing this maneuver and tension to the stoma to be avoided.

3. At last the bowel is to be anchored with interrupted absorbable sutures to the sheath and lastly to the skin.

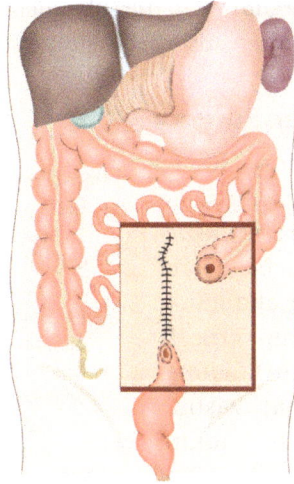

**Fig. 13.2:** End colostomy and mucous fistula

**Table 13.2A:** Indications for colostomy

| Defunctioning loop colostomy | End or loop end colostomy |
|---|---|
| • Lowrectal/coloanal anastomosis | • Abdomino perineal resection |
| • Relief of distal obstruction | • Low anterior resection in patient not suitable for coloanal anastomosis |
| • Rectal trauma/Sphincter injury | • Hartmann's procedure |
| • Fecal incontinence | • Fecal incontinence |
| • Turnbull Blowhole colostomy | • Radiation proctitis |
| • Complex rectovaginal, recto urethral fistula | |
| • Necrotising fasciitis of perineum | |
| • Fournier gangrene | |

It is important to see that stoma protrudes from the skin surface adequately.

Some surgeons prefer to place a polypropelene mesh between the peritonium and the rectus muscle and anchor it so that there is no chance of development of parastomal hernia in future.

In the past, surgeons used to close the lateral space between the lateral side of the bowel and the abdominal wall but there was little evidence to support this, and the technique has fallen into disuse. The abdominal wound is closed and dressed before the colostomy is opened and sutured to the skin.

All layers of the bowel are sutured to the subcuticular tissue or to small bites of the abdominal wall using an absorbable suture such as vicryl.

## End Ileostomy at Open Surgery

The terminal end of closed ileum should be delivered through the stoma opening to the exterior so that the free edge of its mesentery can be sutured to the underside of the abdominal wall along a line running up vertically from the stoma to the falciform ligament so as to prevent twisting. An alternative is to make a tunnel under the peritoneum as described by Goligher, but few surgeons do this now (Figs. 13.3 to 13.5).

Once the abdominal wall is closed and dressed, the ileostomy is opened and sutured in place. They should include the subcuticular tissue of the skin, the seromuscular layer of the ileum at the level of the skin and the full thickness of the ileum at the

**Ileostomy**
- Effluent very corrosive to skin. 1–2 days.
- Output should be "porridgey", 350–600 mL per day.
- Increased/fluid output –infection, diet, drugs
- Obstruction- foods high in cellulose, adhesions, strangulated hernia, stenosis
- Stoma edematous, cramps, fluid effluent then ceases
- Imodium
- High output stoma 800 ml to 2 litres, TPN, electrolyte replacement
- Loop ileostomy can be difficult to manage due to its odd shape, mucus from distal part
- High output ileostomy – electrolyte drinks, TPN, appliance type
- Chemotherapy treatment- increasing stoma activity, skin more sensitive, reduced feeling in patient's fingers

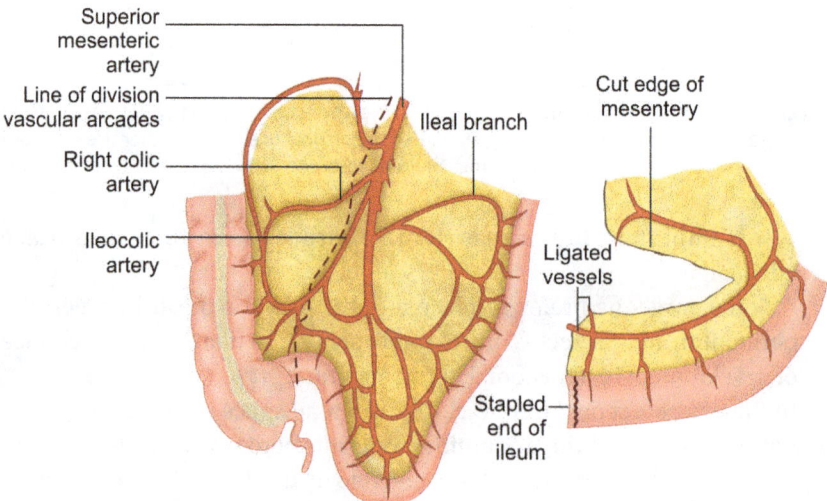

**Fig. 13.3:** End ileostomy

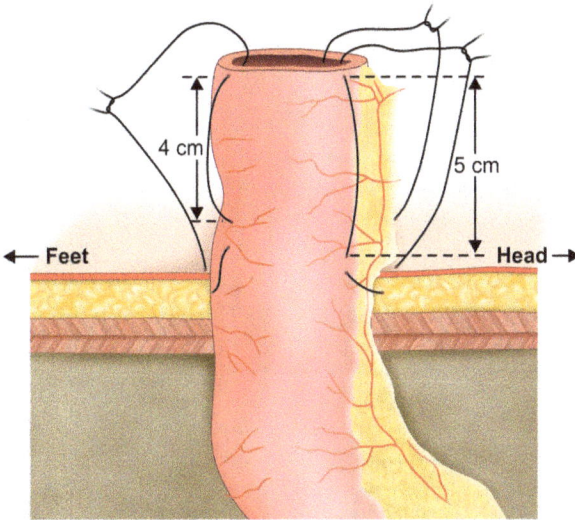

**Fig. 13.4:** Eversion of stoma and suturing to abdominal wall

opened end. These sutures are held in clips and then tensioned together so as to achieve formation of the spout. It is important that the seromuscular stitch is not too deep in order to prevent the formation of a fistula at the level of the skin.

## Loop Ileostomy at Open Surgery (Fig. 13.6)

1. To perform a loop ileostomy, a segment of ileum should be marked with a diathermy or sutures to recognise proximal and distal segments of ileum.
2. This segment of ileum forming the stoma should be mobile and adequately away from the ileocecal junction.
3. One should know that the opening of the anterior abdominal wall at the site of stoma is larger, than for an end ileostomy.
4. The segment of the ileum can be brought out from the abdomen to the exterior by grasping with Babkock forceps or a traction through a catheter or guaze tape through an opening made at the mesentric border close to the bowel. Then the opening of the abdominal wall is closed.

The ileum is cut open transversely near the skin on the distal non-functioning site so that a projecting everted stoma is created on the functioning side.

Then absorbable sutures are used to suture the ileal end of the stoma to the abdominal wall in an interrupted fashion. A single piece ileostomy bag is fitted for draining the stoma.

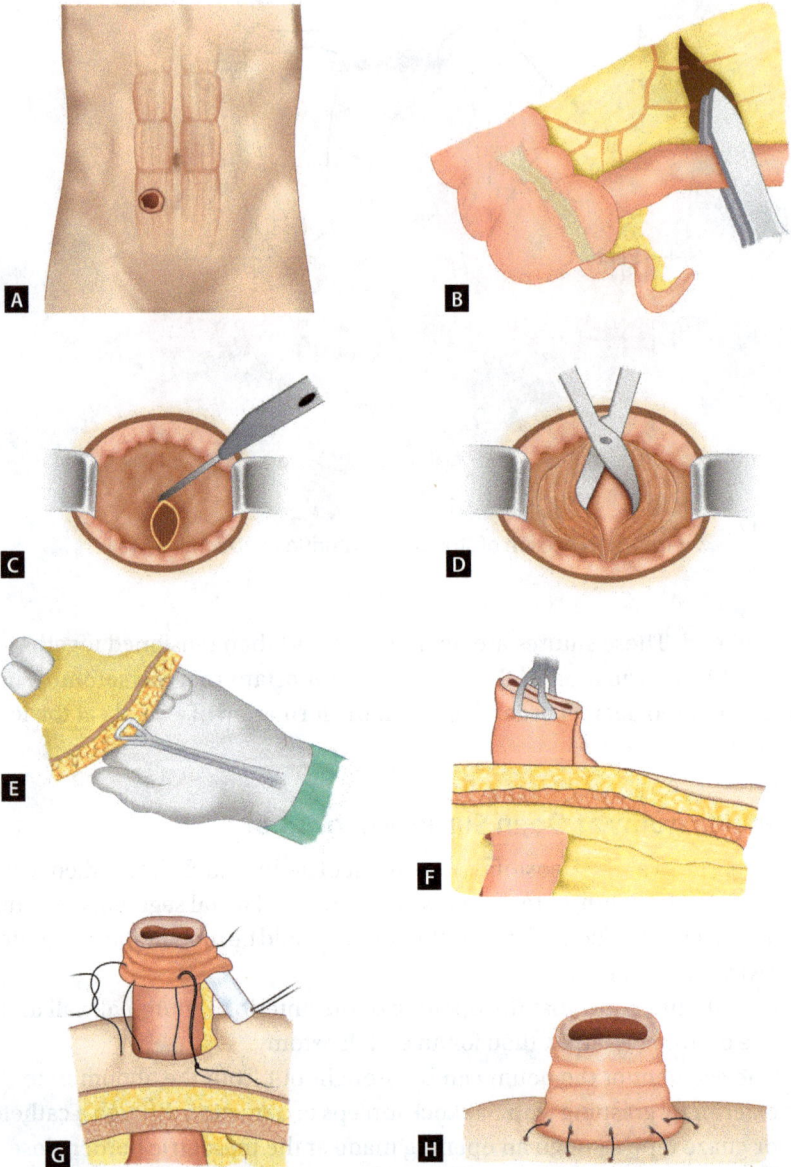

**Figs. 13.5A to H:** Formation of end Ileostomy. (A) Site of stoma marking; (B) Division of distal ileum with GIA stapler; (C) Cruciate incision in anterior rectus sheath following excision of circle of skin; (D) Splitting of rectus muscle; (E) Ensuring opening accommodates two fingers: (F) Gentle delivery of end of ileum through abdominal wall with Babcock forceps; (G) Eversion of the end ileostomy with Langenbeck forceps and suturing to abdominal wall; (H) Completed end ileostomy

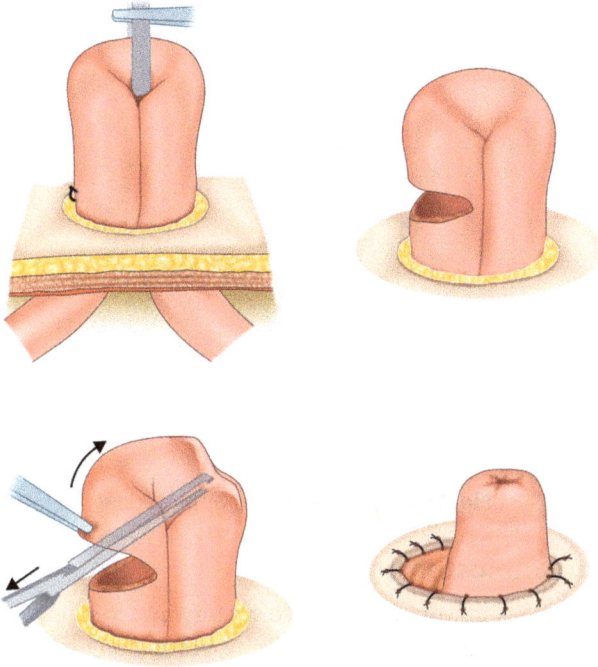

**Fig. 13.6:** Loop ileostomy

## Trephine or Blowhole Transverse Colostomy

Trephine or Blowhole transverse colostomy is performed as an emergency procedure when there is a complete obstruction of the distal colon or rectum.

This method can be approached by open, laparoscopic or colonoscopy assisted methods (Fig. 13.7).

This is a short-term procedure to achieve fecal diversion when there is a serious colorectal emergency like toxic mega colon and pelvic malignancies.

This is performed by making a 3 cm incision over the abdominal wall in midline over the transverse colon. The incision is carried down to the fascia and entered into the abdomen.

The distended transverse colon is identified and anchored with fixation sutures and secured to the peritoneum and fascia, thus preventing the spillage of contents into the abdomen.

A transverse colostomy is created by incising the colon with a sharp knife and is matured, then sutured to the skin with interrupted sutures. A colostomy bag is applied over the stoma and secured.

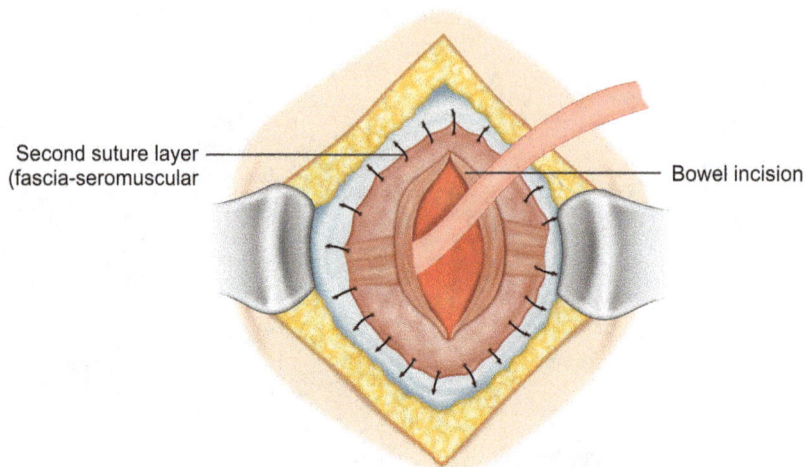

**Fig. 13.7:** Trephine colostomy procedure

## Laparoscopic Colostomy

The latest advances in Minimal invasive surgery involve creation of a stoma by the use of laparoscopic surgery. The operative technique is identical like siting the stoma in general, besides performing the surgery by key hole techniques.

The surgery is begun by creating pneumoperitoneum and then placing multiple ports.

Then the steps of surgery are the same like open technique in terms of identification of the colon, site for stoma, mobilisation of colon and exteriorization of colon for creating the stoma outside the abdomen (Fig. 13.8).

Then the loop is secured with a colostomy rod or a catheter avoiding torsion of mesentry or bleeding. Pneumoperitoneum is reversed and the stoma is created and appliances placed.

## Laparoscopic Ileostomy (Fig. 13.9)

Patient is placed in supine position and after creation of a pneumoperitoneum under anaesthesia,Ports are inserted and ileum is mobilised away from Ileocecal junction and the segment is brought out of the abdominal wall at the site of stoma and secured to the skin and fascia with sutures. Then the ileostomy is matured and a stoma appliance is fitted.

## Principles of Surgery for Urinary Conduit (Figs. 13.10 to 13.13)

The surgical technique consists of choosing a long segment of small intestine to allow stoma to be constructed at the level of the abdominal wall and still

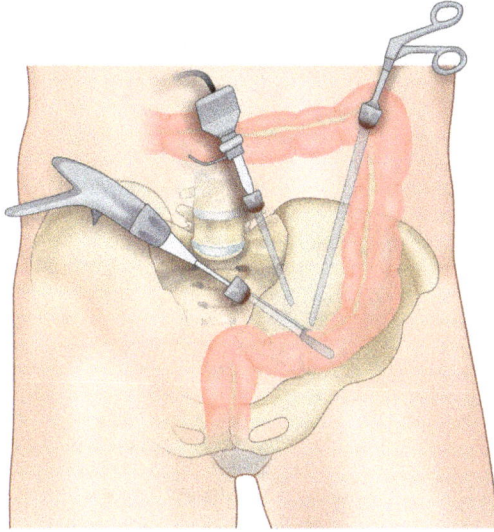

**Fig. 13.8:** Orientation of Laparoscopic instruments—Colon resection

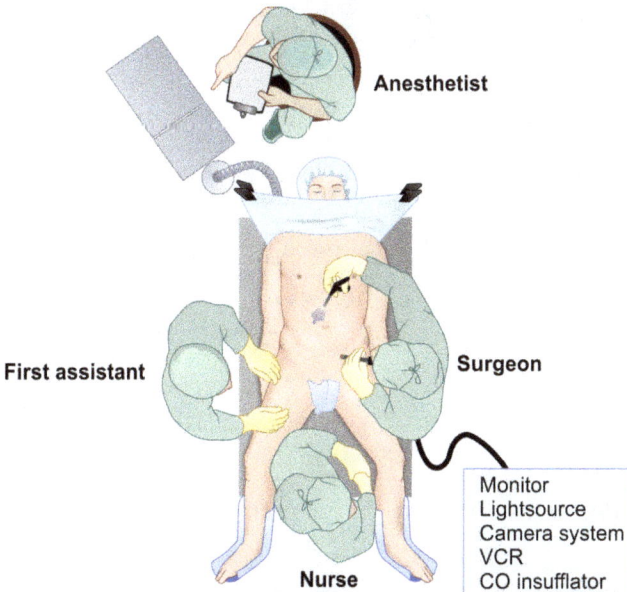

Anesthetist

First assistant

Surgeon

Nurse

Monitor
Lightsource
Camera system
VCR
CO insufflator

**Fig. 13.9:** Preparation for Laparoscopic Ileostomy

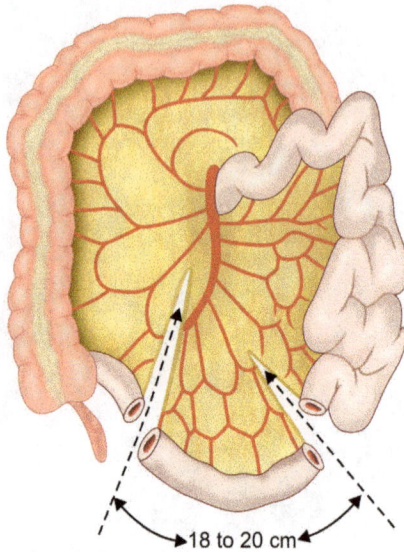

**Fig. 13.10:** An 18 to 20 cm segment of distal ileum is taken out in continuity with its blood supply

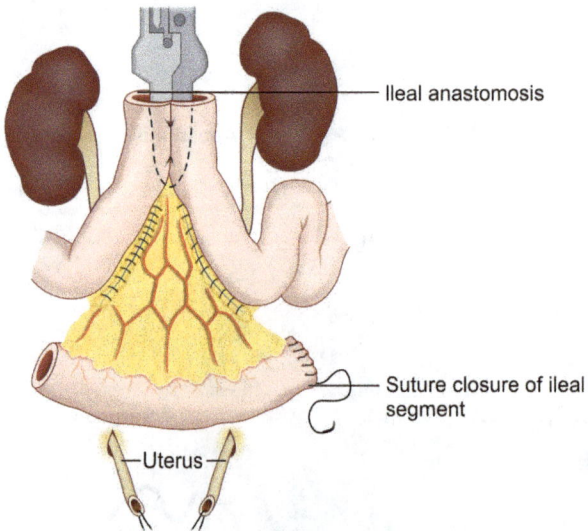

**Fig. 13.11:** Intestinal continuity restored and the conduit is located posteriorly

allow the proximal end to reach close enough to the retro peritoneum to prevent tension on the uretero intestinal anastomosis. Usually 18 to 20 cm of intestine is enough but this may be modified if there is a short mesentry or obese abdominal wall.

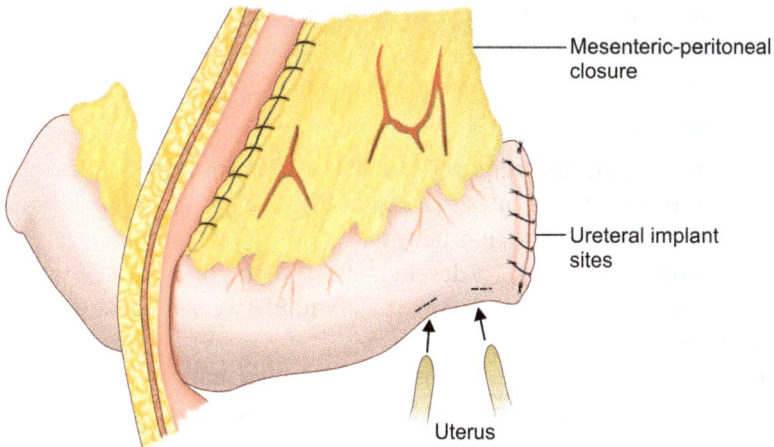

Mesenteric-peritoneal closure

Ureteral implant sites

Uterus

**Fig. 13.12:** The ureteral conduit anastomosis completed

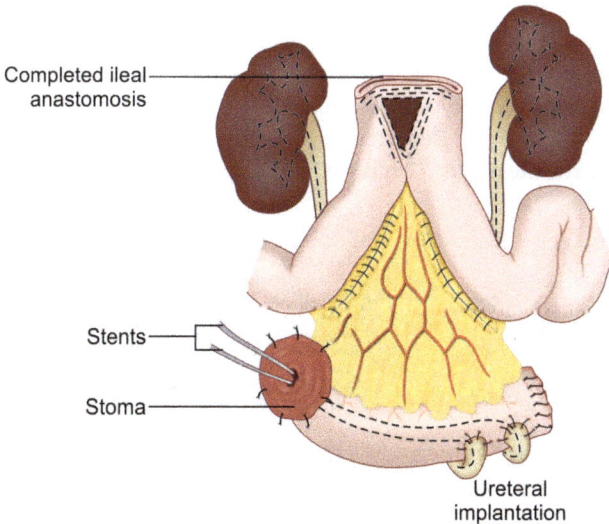

Completed ileal anastomosis

Stents

Stoma

Ureteral implantation

**Fig. 13.13:** Stents are placed through the completed ureteral anastomosis

After choosing a segment of small intestine the mesentry at the distal point is incised and continued to transect the mesentery converging to both ends of the intestine preserving its blood supply.

It is positioned posterior to the restored intestine. The ileoileal anastomosis is completed with sutures or staplers. The selected conduit is cleaned off its intestinal contents and its proximal end is closed. Closure should be done with absorbable sutures.

An opening is made in the abdominal wall to construct the stoma.

The ureteral anastomosis is performed with the conduit in its final position at the proximal site and stents are placed.

## ■ OSTOMY CLOSURE AND TIME

- A second operation required in case of temporary ileostomies and colostomies to restore intestinal continuity
- 17% morbidity and 0.4% mortality rate
- 4% require laparotomy, 7% develop bowel obstruction
- Studies suggest safety of selective early (within 3 weeks) and late strategies depending on clinical circumstances
- Early closure associated with reduced hospital stay, bowel obstruction and medical complications but increased wound infection rates.

## ■ BIBLIOGRAPHY

1. http://www.seminarscolonrectalsurgery.com/article/S1043-1489(08)00043-2/fulltext
2. https://www.ncbi.nlm.nih.gov/pubmed/22873030.
3. Intestinal stomas: Indications,Management and Complications
4. Laparoscopic Ileostomy and Colostomy
5. Martin ST, Vogel JD. Department of Colorectal surgery,Digestive Disease Institute, The Cleaveland Clinic,9500Euclid Avenue, Cleveland OH 44195, USA.

# Role of Enterostomal Nurse

## ■ PREOPERATIVE CONSIDERATIONS

Preoperative preparation is a very important step in providing a good quality of life. It involves not only the successful management of the underlying disease of the patient but also a good functioning stoma.

For achieving this successful goal of providing a stoma with a good quality life to the patient, Enterostomal nurse plays a very important role.

There are number of issues which are to be understood for the success or failure towards ostomy.

They are, understanding the patients' attitude towards ostomy creation, for example: fear, misunderstanding, misinformation, anatomical considerations, other health problems or physical disabilities.

> **Patient impact**
> - Stoma formation and stoma complications can effect the physical, psychological, sexuality and social well-being of the patient
> - Loss of self-esteem
> - Change in body image
> - Loss of confidence
> - Social recluse
> - Affecting work, relationships, social activities/holidays
> - Regular support especially early in recovery period is vital

## Attitude of the Patient (Table 14.1)

Most of the patients consider creating a stoma in them is worse than being dead. Hence, it is very important to make them understand and counsel them in order to remove the fear in their mind. This fear can be mitigated by educating the patient with the available resources.

The patient nurse has a very high responsibility to address all the psychological issues preventing the patient in creation of stoma.

There are many ways in dealing with the patient in alleging the fear:
- Enterostomal nurse can involve the stoma organization volunteers to visit the patient and convince them about the acceptance of stoma.
- The enterostomal nurse along with the surgeon is also responsible for treating the stoma, can jointly talk to the patient and discuss about the importance of stoma and educate the patient about the appliances available and its usage in day-to-day life.
- The enterostomal nurse has to reassure the patient that their sexual relationship would remain unaffected.

**Table 14.1:** Gender based concerns about stoma

| Male patients' concern | Female patients' concern |
|---|---|
| Do I have to change my profession? | Will this hinder my daily routine? |
| Will my family members and relatives accept me? | Can I enter the kitchen and cook? |
| Can I continue with my fitness routine? | Will I be allowed to enter pooja room or places of worship? |
| Am I fit for married life? (If married) am I fit for sexual life? | Am I fit for married life? (If married) am I fit for sexual life? |
| Can I travel as usual? | Can I continue with my fitness routine? |
| Do I have to disclose this to relatives and friends? | Do I have to disclose this to relatives and friends? |
| Will I be accepted in my friends' circle? | Can I try out modern outfits? |

- The enterostomal nurse should address the patient regarding the other activities like participation in sports swimming, wearing special clothing and dietary habits. Such counseling is a very important step in achieving a good quality of life for the patient and decreases the complications following stoma surgery.

## Anatomical Considerations

It is a very important step to select the site over body for selection of stoma.

The stoma site should be marked preoperatively by the enterostomal nurse in such a way that the patient is able to change positions and demonstrate his/her ability to see and work with that site.

Enterostomal nurse has to give consideration to all the usual landmarks including the costal margins, umbilicus, waist line and groins. In addition, scars of previous surgery, skin folds should be identified to avoid placement of the stoma.

The site should be marked with patient standing and sit on the edge of a table.

The ostomy triangle should be identified which is bordered by the umbilicus, the anterior superior iliac spine and the pubic symphisus.

The stoma should be placed through the rectus and the site of stoma is no closer than 5 cm to any bony prominence or fold crease or scar.

Patient should be able to confirm and touch and see the site of stoma while standing or lying down.

It is important to select the site below the hip line to allow more flexibility in clothing selection. Patients' confidence will be boosted after wearing the clothing, covering the pouching system. It is important to wear loose clothing above the applicance.

## Special Considerations

- *Physical challenges*: Those who cannot visualize or touch the stoma should be given preference in placing of stoma.
- The placement should be done to facilitate the caretakers' needs in the management of stoma. So it should be placed higher or lower site where it is used to be otherwise selected.
- For wheelchair patients, the stoma site should be marked when they are sitting in the wheelchair, with the patients' preference to see and manage them.

Those patients who are using brace or other devices for the support of the back, the stoma site should be selected to avoid their contact with the appliances.

## Other Special Problems

In case of cancer patients who have history of radiation or about to get radiation, it is better to avoid placing the stoma within the radiation field.

In severely obese patients, visualization of the stoma may be difficult by the patient when he/she sitting or lying down. In such patients, it is ideal to place the stoma at a higher level.

Patients who need double stoma like urostomy and normal stoma with pouching belts, it is better to have them located on the opposite sides of the abdomen with the urostomy at a higher level.

*The general principles of selecting the stoma are :*
- They should pass through the rectus muscle.
- In midline stoma they should pass through Linea alba.
- They should be positioned 6 cm away from the costal margin or iliac crest or any other bony prominence.
- Avoid prior scars or prior stoma sites. Rarely it can be brought through the surgical wound when no other options are available.
- It is necessary for the patients to wear the stoma kit for 24 to 48 hours before the surgery to access the acceptability of its position.

## ■ PREOPERATIVE COUNSELING

It is necessary to counsel the patient one week before the surgery regarding the stoma.

Counseling a male and a female ostomate is different. It is better to counsel the ostomates through the Ostomy visitors who are of the same gender.

It is better to counsel not only the patient regarding the stoma but also the spouse or the close caretaker who are going to manage the stoma.

For illiterate patients, emotional soothing through a lot of anecdotes are needed to counsel them.

Confidentiality is to be maintained during counseling.

Listening to patients before counseling is a must.

Booklets, pamphlets and websites are the alternative sources to counsel the literate patients. In case of male patients, attention should be given more if he is the bread winner of the family.

## ■ POSTOPERATIVE ROLE

Postoperatively the enterostomal therapy (ET) nurse instructs the patients and family in:

- Ostomy care
- Dietary and fluid alterations
- Ways to incorporate ostomy management into patients' life.

The ET nurse also provides long-term follow-up care in outpatient settings. Such care includes ongoing counseling education and surveillance for complication requiring medical intervention.

ET nurses can recommend appropriate measures to prevent and manage skin break down that is related to immobility, friable skin, and incontinence and/or radiation therapy. They can also assist in correcting or containing fecal or urinary incontinence and in cost effective management of draining wounds and fistulas.

In the immediate postoperative period the stoma should be checked regularly when the patient is in recovery or on the ward.

There is a clear drainable bag placed over the stoma and one can view the stoma through the bag, the color and the discharge of the liquid from the stoma into the bag.

*The following postoperative features of stoma should be seen:*

- Color
- Output
- Rod in place
- Skin condition
- Stoma spout and size
- Sutures

### Color of the Stoma

The color of the healthy stoma (Figs. 14.1A to C) is pink to bright red. A pale colour stoma indicates low hemoglobin, a dusky stoma as purple or very dark red in color may indicate lack of blood supply to the stoma.

A black necrotic stoma indicates no blood supply to the stoma.

The ET nurse should inform the surgical team if there are any concerns regarding the color of the stoma.

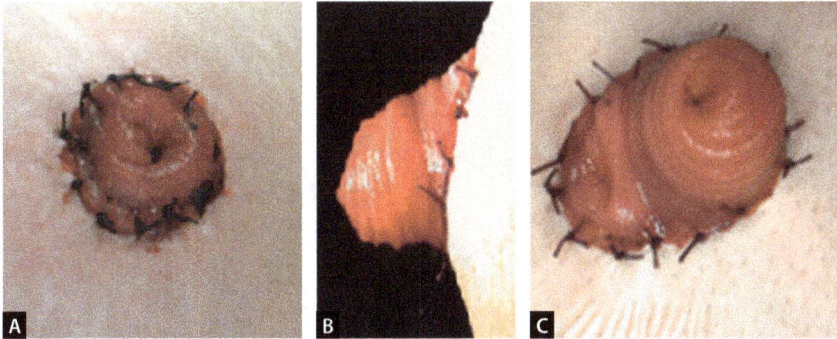

**Figs. 14.1A to C:** Healthy stoma. (A) End colostomy; (B) End ileostomy; (C) Loop ileostomy

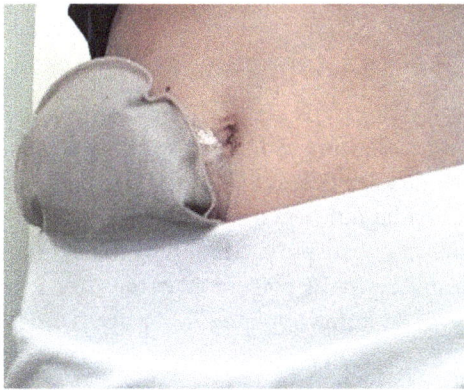

**Fig. 14.2:** Stoma filled with flatus

## Output

The first sign of functioning of the bowel is filling up of stoma with the flatus (Fig. 14.2). Subsequently there will be output of liquid in the bag which may vary from serosanginos or green in color indicating bile. These features are seen after about 2 to 3 days post surgery.

The output from the Ileostomy is gruel like (a thin liquid food of oatmeal or other meal boiled in the milk or water) measuring 600 to 800 mL in 24 hours.

The output of colostomy resembles a formed motion. A urostomy starts functioning immediately with urine.

## Rod in Place (Fig. 14.3)

A rod is a hard plastic tube that is place under the loop of the stoma. This plastic tube is usually left under the loop for a period of 1 week to 10 days and is removed based on surgeon's instruction.

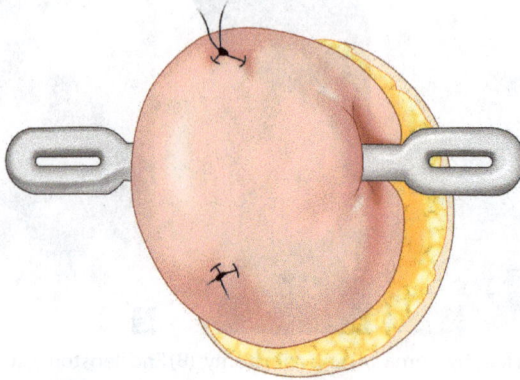

**Fig. 14.3:** Rod in place under the stoma to prevent it from pulling under the skin

### Skin Condition (Figs. 14.4, 14.5 and Flowchart 14.1)

The condition of the skin can be seen only when the stoma bag is changed. Skin complications can develop soon after surgery and can harm the patient around the stoma if leakage occurs. This may cause embarrassment, loss of confidence and poor adaptation to life with stoma.

A leaking stoma may cause excoriation of the skin around the stoma, thereby causing problems in the placement of the stoma appliances.

Sometimes allergy to stoma appliance or its accessories may rarely cause skin complication.

### Stoma Spout and Size (Fig. 14.9)

The ideal length of the stoma should be between 3 and 5 cm. The spout should protrude from the skin sufficiently to avoid skin excoriation. After surgery the stoma will be oedematous. But over a period of 6 to 8 weeks it reduces to an adaptable size.

### Sutures Surrounding the Stoma

There may be sutures around the junction of skin and the stoma. This may take from days to weeks to dissolve and fall. Patients should be made aware of such things.

### ■ APPLIANCES (FIG. 14.10)

Patients have many choices for the appliances to fit into the stoma. They are divided into one and two piece products which can be closed or drainable. For ileostomy, the appliance has a drain at the bottom for the patients to empty it.

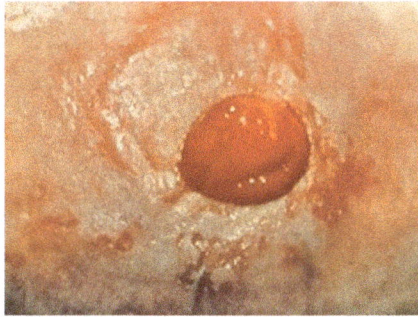

**Fig. 14.4:** Irritant dermatitis

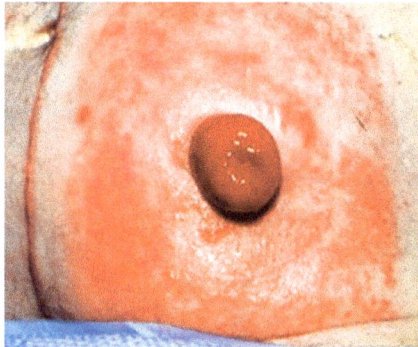

**Fig. 14.5:** Allergic contat dermatitis

**Flowchart 14.1:** Skin complications—Types, causes and management

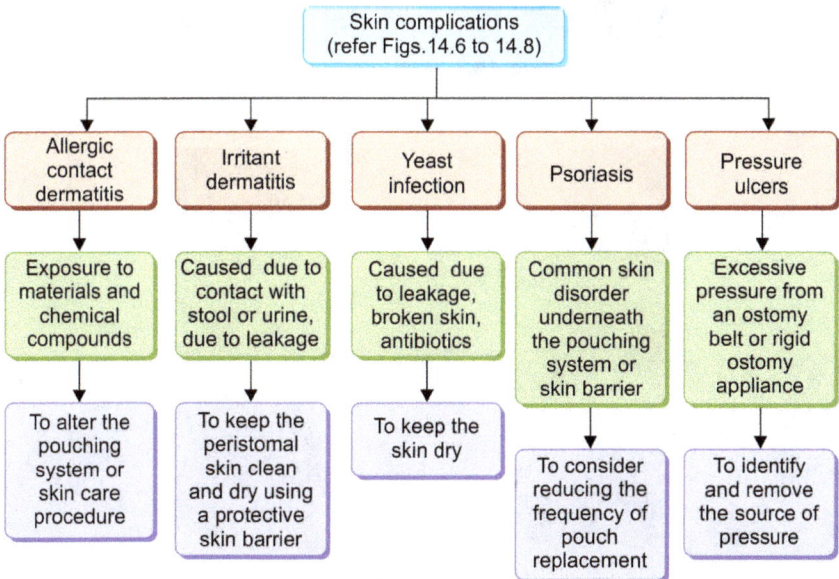

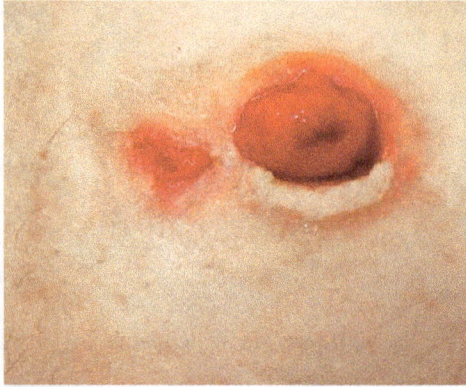

**Fig. 14.6:** Pressure ulcer

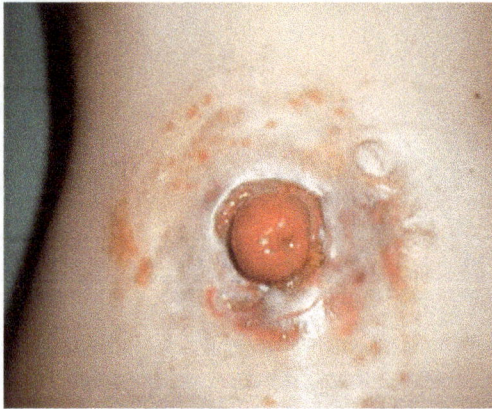

**Fig. 14.7:** Yeast infection

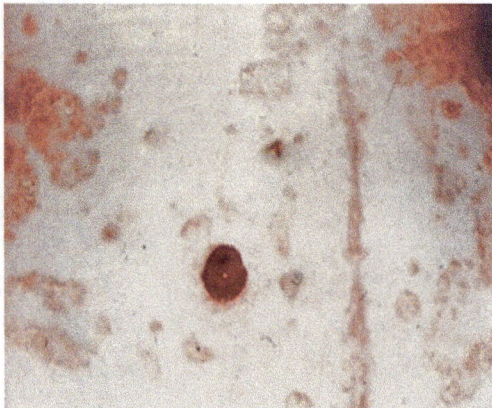

**Fig. 14.8:** Psoriasis

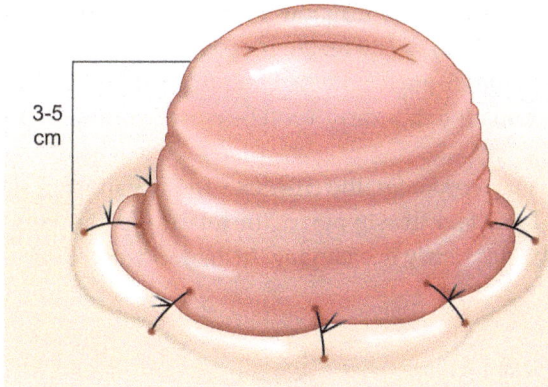

**Fig. 14.9:** Healthy Stoma

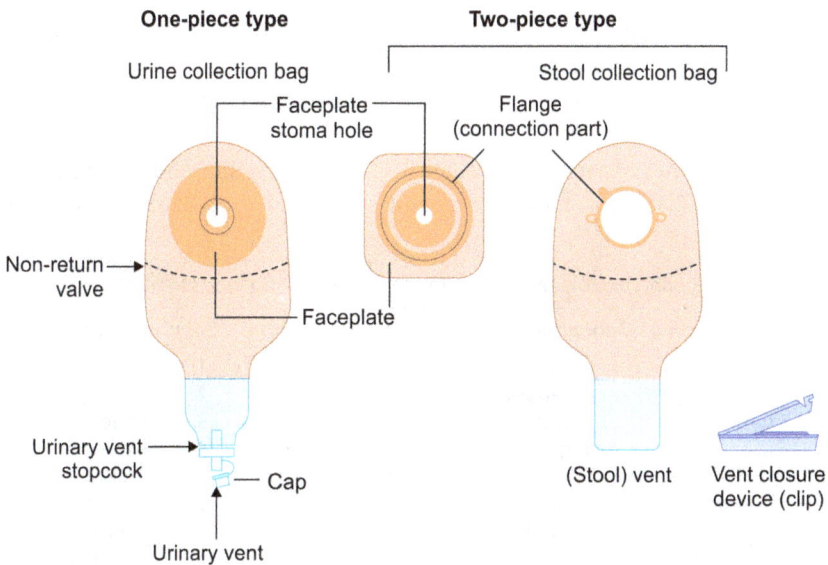

**Fig. 14.10:** Stoma appliances

For urostomy, there is a tap at the bottom. These appliances can be changed daily or every 2 or 3 days depending on the patients' lifestyle, skin condition, the wear and tear time of the appliance.

For colostomy, a closed appliance is more appropriate which can be detached and drained.

## PSYCHOLOGICAL SUPPORT

The creation of a stoma in patients' body can raise many issues to the patient like acceptance, fear, anxiety about body image and body functions.

When the patient wakes up after surgery and notices the stoma with appliance, most of them would feel depressed to see alteration of their body image. However, the ET nurse and the attending surgeon should reassure the patient, if the stoma is temporary, it will be closed getting back the patient to normal.

If the stoma is permanent, the ET nurse and the surgeon should comfort the patient and also seek the support of the relatives of the patient to take care emotionally and physically in changing the bag and attending to the patients' requirement.

## ■ DIET (TABLE 14.2)

The diet is a very important factor to the ostomates as is for the rest of the population. It is better to depend on the home made foods and avoid junk foods.

Carbohydrate foods such as bread, rice, potatoes should make 1/3 of the diet. Fruits and vegetables could be taken in smaller proportions.

Protein foods such as meat, fish, egg white, beans and pulses are essential for maintaining strength and immune function.

Milk and dairy foods that are good source of protein and calcium with minerals and vitamins could be taken in reasonable proportions. Yoghurt

**Table14.2:** Showing trouble managing and troubleshooting foods for ostomates

| Stoma obstructing | Odor producing | Increased/loose stool | Gas producing |
|---|---|---|---|
| 1. Apple peel | 1. Asparagus | 1. Apple juice | 1. Alcoholic beverage |
| 2. Raw cabbage | 2. Baked bean | 2. Alcoholic | 2. Beans |
| 3. Corn | 3. Brocolli | beverage | 3. Cabbage |
| 4. Coconut | 4. Egg | 3. Bran cereals | 4. Cauliflower |
| 5. Dried fruits | 5. Fish | 4. Cooked cabbage | 5. Cucumber |
| 6. Mushrooms | 6. Garlic | 5. Fresh fruits | 6. Carbonated drinks |
| 7. Orange | 7. Onion | 6. Milk | 7. Chewing gums |
| 8. Pineapple | 8. Peanut butter | 7. Prunes | 8. Dairy products |
| 9. Nuts | 9. Strong cheese | 8. Raisins | 9. Milk/Nuts |
| 10. Popcorn | 10. Some vitamins | 9. Spices | 10. Onions |
| Constipation relief | Odor control | Loose stool control | Reducing flatus |
| 1. Coffee warm/ hot | 1. Butter milk | 1. Apple sauce | 1. Cranberry juice |
| 2. Fruits and vegetables cooked | 2. Cranberry juice | 2. Boiled rice | 2. Butter milk |
|  | 3. Tomato juice | 3. White bread | 3. Peppermint oil |
|  | 4. Yoghurt | 4. Potato | **Color changes** |
| 3. Water | 5. Peppermint oil | 5. Pasta | 1. Food color |
| 4. Mild laxatives |  | 6. Marsh mallows | 2. Iron pills |
| 5. Fresh fruits |  |  | 3. Strawberry |
| 6. Fruit juices |  |  | 4. Asparagus |
|  |  |  | 5. Beets |
|  |  |  | 6. Tomato sauce |

and butter milk are an excellent source of lactobacillus and yeast which helps in maintaining intestinal bacterial flora.

Fats and sugar can be taken at a smaller proportion. Foods with high fiber content should be avoided in the case of Ileostomy patients. Ileostomy patients are advised to take more minerals as diarrhea is more common.

*Indian millets and curd rice are always safe.*

### ■ FOODS TO AVOID

Beans, peas, unripe banana and potato should not be consumed excessively as they contain sugar and starch which can escape digestion and enter the colon where they are fermented to produce gas. Beer and fizzy drinks may also increase the amount of flatulence.

Very spicy foods can irritate the digestive system and cause loose motions. Artificial sweeteners can also cause loose motions.

### ■ LIFESTYLE MODIFICATIONS OF PATIENTS WITH OSTOMY

The ET nurse has to visit the ostomy patient after discharge from hospital to find out how they are recovering and when they can resume a normal lifestyle.
- They are encouraged to mobilize as their tolerance allows.
- It is advised not to undertake heavy lifting or activities for 3 months after surgery.
- As far as driving is concerned (patients can start sooner they are able to do) it is advised to start once they are confident with walking and their strength has increased to perform such activities.
  Usually it takes a minimum of 2 weeks after discharge but it can be considerably longer.
- Work and exercises can be started after about 2 to 4 weeks once they are able to perform daily routines.
- Holidays can be taken after 3 months once the ostomates are confident of flying but should remember to have their appliances in their hand luggage and it is necessary to take a travel advice from the ET nurse.

## Diet (Fig. 14.11)

Dietary guidelines should be recommended by the treating doctor and ET nurse to the ostomy patients.

If the patient has ileostomy the following advices are to be taken:
- They should drink 8 to 10 glasses of liquids a day.
- To limit the intake of caffeine and alcohol
- To limit foods like high fiber and high sugar content products.
- If one feels bloating and pain after eating certain food, it is better to avoid them.

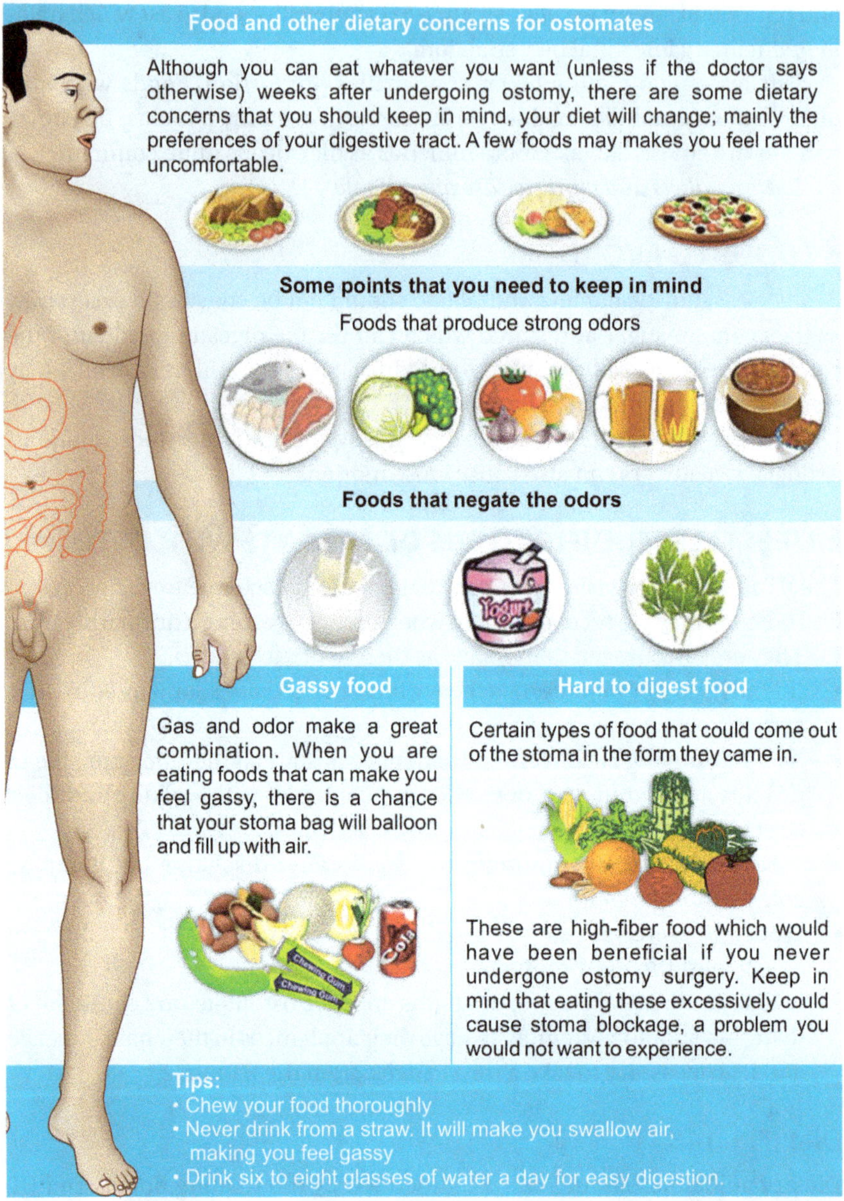
Food and other dietary concerns for ostomates
Although you can eat whatever you want (unless if the doctor says otherwise) weeks after undergoing ostomy, there are some dietary concerns that you should keep in mind, your diet will change; mainly the preferences of your digestive tract. A few foods may makes you feel rather uncomfortable.
Some points that you need to keep in mind
Foods that produce strong odors
Foods that negate the odors
Yogurt
Gassy food
Gas and odor make a great combination. When you are eating foods that can make you feel gassy, there is a chance that your stoma bag will balloon and fill up with air.
Chewing Gum
Chewing Gum
Cola
Hard to digest food
Certain types of food that could come out of the stoma in the form they came in.
These are high-fiber food which would have been beneficial if you never undergone ostomy surgery. Keep in mind that eating these excessively could cause stoma blockage, a problem you would not want to experience.
Tips:
• Chew your food thoroughly
• Never drink from a straw. It will make you swallow air, making you feel gassy
• Drink six to eight glasses of water a day for easy digestion.

**Fig. 14.11:** Dietary concerns for Ostomates

- Certain gas producing foods like cabbage, broccoli, carbonated beverages and chewing gum should be avoided.
- If one feels constipated it is advised to drink more liquids, eat foods with high fiber content such as fruits, vegetables and bran.
- Better to walk around.
- If the patient has ileostomy, better to avoid laxative.

## Medication (Table 14.3)

An ostomate must consider carefully before taking any drugs either through prescription or over-the-counter. In case of prescribed drugs, the Ostomates should inform the general practitioner (GP) about their prevailing condition to avoid side effects which are specific to the ostomates.

**Table 14.3:** The following table focuses on the different drugs and their effects on the stoma

| *Drugs* | *Colostomy* | *Ileostomy* | *Urostomy* |
|---|---|---|---|
| **Antacids** (Gelusil/Digene) | Products containing aluminium may cause constipation | Products containing magnesium may cause diarrhea | Products containing calcium may cause calcium stones |
| **Antibiotics** | May destroy normal flora | May lead to diarrhoea and risk of dehydration (e.g. ampicilin, cephalosporin, sulphonamides) | Usually no problem |
| **Contraceptives** | Usually no problem | Birth control pills may not be absorbed. There may be a possible need to use other birth control measures | Usually no problem |
| **Steroids** | Sodium retention. Possibility of fungal infection due to suppression of immune system | Sodium retention. Possibility of fungal infection due to suppression of immune system | Sodium retention. Possibility of fungal infection due to suppression of immune system |
| **Diuretics** | Usually no problem | May cause electrolyte imbalance | Will increase urine flow. May cause electrolyte imbalance |
| Non-steroidal anti-inflammatory agents **(NSAIDs)** | May cause bleeding from stomach or duodenum-gastric distress. Do not take on an empty stomach | May cause bleeding from stomach or duodenum-gastric distress. Do not take on an empty stomach | May cause bleeding from stomach or duodenum-gastric distress. Do not take on an empty stomach |
| **Vitamins** | Liquid form is best. B Complex may cause odor | Liquid form is best. B Complex may cause odor. Vitamin B12 is the best by injection or nasal spray. Not absorbed well by oral route | B Complex may cause odor. Tablet/capsule is okay. |

The problem of taking medication in an ileostomy patient is that the tablets and the capsules which may be coated or time release type may not give better absorption or benefit. The best choice of medication for an ileostomy patient is uncoated tablets or liquid form.

## ■ DAY-TO-DAY ACTIVITY

The ostomates should not feel that they are handicapped in their lives. They are equally capable of leading a normal life like any other healthy individual.

### At Work

Returning to work is a good way to get back to normal routine and working again can make the ostomate feel good about themselves. They should arrive early to their workplace so that they can empty their bags/change the pouches that they feel comfortable at work without being inconvenient to others and also not wasting their productive work hours.

It is better for an ostomate to come prepared with the home made food which can be tolerated and does not cause any harm to the digestive system. It is also advised to avoid frequent snacking and eating shared food with the colleagues which might sometimes cause disturbance in their digestion. It is advisable for the ostomates to carry extra pouches and medications that may be necessary.

It is better to talk to the employer regarding the ostomy so that the ostomates can be given appropriate work schedule. An ostomate who is nervous about caring for ostomy at work can talk to the doctor or an ostomy nurse who could guide properly. At work, mere worrying about oneself and their ostomy may not bring the best out of them.

### Clothing

There is no limit to clothing for an ostomate. However, the stoma location may make some clothes uncomfortable. It is better to avoid tight clothing, waist bands or belts that may press upon the stoma. It is better to experiment different styles of clothing and then choose the comfortable one.

In India, where the clothing pattern is different as compared to the Western countries, the pouch can be hidden underneath the petticoat and could be covered by saree.

### Showering, Bathing, and Swimming

Patient with ostomy can take bath with the pouching system on or off. However, patient with ileostomy should keep the pouch on during shower due to possible drainage of bowel movements while taking bath. One can prevent the leakage by putting waterproof tape around the edges of the waffer. Sometimes patients can provide improvised plastic cover tied over the pouching system from getting it wet.

## Sports Activity

If you are a sports person who wants to continue with your hobby/passion you may continue to do so but with prior precautions.

You will need time after your surgery to heal and recover and eventually gain strength and stamina to enjoy your sports.

The main concern about sports activity is injury to the stoma and its appliances causing leakage of the waste or urine leading to embarassment. Hence, one has to take prior precautionary measures to bolster and protect the stoma and its appliances with special appliances like belt or binder to hold your stoma bag in place.

Such products are available with the stoma suppliers in different patterns or else one can improvise according to their convenience. It is better to avoid contact sports, since it involves a lot of potential for injury. But it is wise to ask your doctor or ostomy nurse before pursuing any sports and take their advice.

Ostomates can pursue swimming with passion, only thing is that they have to take precautionary measures to protect the stoma and prevent any leakage.

It is wise to empty your ostomy bag before you embark on any sports activity. It is sometimes worthy to get an opinion from a trusted colleague/close friend/loved ones about the visibility of your bag under your clothes and correct it.

## Travel (Fig. 14.12)

Having a stoma is not an obstacle to travel but there are some issues one should be aware of before travel.

### Traveling by Road (Fig. 14.13)

It is not advisable to drive immediately after surgery because the driver may not be able to focus on driving because of the concern over their stoma. Seat belt in the car can be worn without pressure on the stoma. Certain special accessories are available for the seat belts which can be used as a replacement.

It is better to take shorter trips in the initial stages and build your confident levels. It is wise to take advice from your stoma therapy nurse or the surgeon who operated you before you go for the travel. Keep your supplies at cool place, because hot weather can affect the adhesives on the pouches.

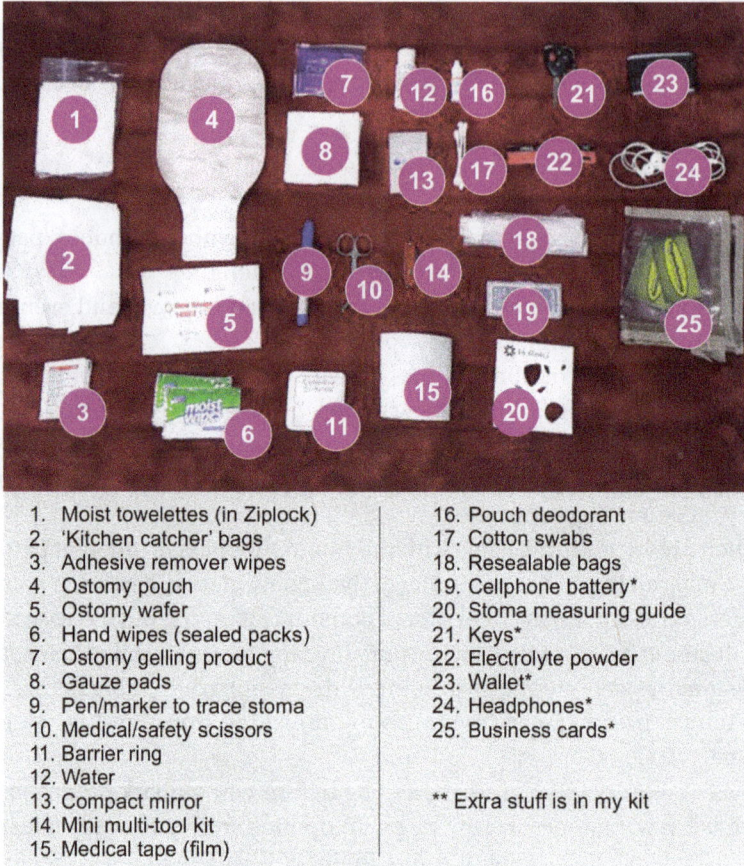

1. Moist towelettes (in Ziplock)
2. 'Kitchen catcher' bags
3. Adhesive remover wipes
4. Ostomy pouch
5. Ostomy wafer
6. Hand wipes (sealed packs)
7. Ostomy gelling product
8. Gauze pads
9. Pen/marker to trace stoma
10. Medical/safety scissors
11. Barrier ring
12. Water
13. Compact mirror
14. Mini multi-tool kit
15. Medical tape (film)
16. Pouch deodorant
17. Cotton swabs
18. Resealable bags
19. Cellphone battery*
20. Stoma measuring guide
21. Keys*
22. Electrolyte powder
23. Wallet*
24. Headphones*
25. Business cards*

** Extra stuff is in my kit

**Fig. 14.12:** Ostomy travel kit

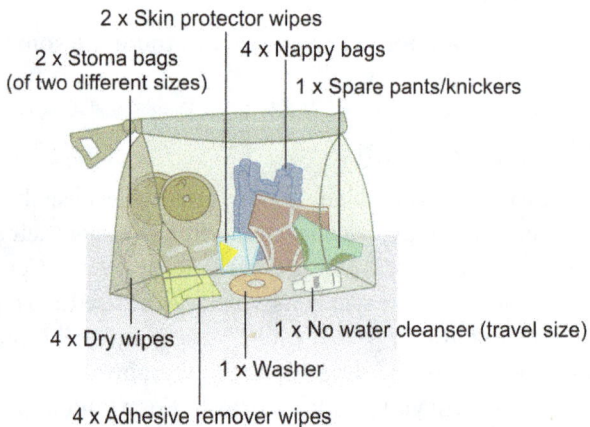

2 x Skin protector wipes
2 x Stoma bags
(of two different sizes)
4 x Nappy bags
1 x Spare pants/knickers
4 x Dry wipes
1 x No water cleanser (travel size)
1 x Washer
4 x Adhesive remover wipes

**Fig. 14.13:** Day-to-day travel supplies with a stoma bag

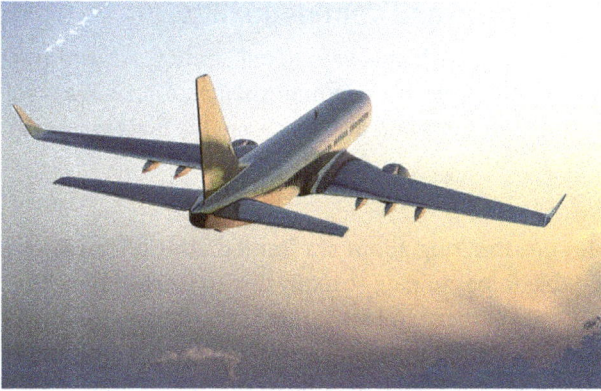

**Fig. 14.14:** Traveling by air

One must prepare a checklist before embarking on travel and gather all the items. The list include pouches, wipes, and filters, disposable bags, doctor's certificates, appropriate clothes, prescribed drugs, and contact numbers of the surgeon, ET nurse and close relatives. It is better to carry enough supplies of all the items in the checklist when you plan for travel.

### Consideration While Traveling by Air (Fig. 14.14)

It is advised not to travel by air within the first 6 weeks following surgery because of increased risk of deep vein thrombosis (DVT). It is better to keep your supplies in your main luggage and also in your hand luggage to meet their demands during an emergency.

Base plates to be cut and kept ready to use since scissors are not permitted to be carried during travel.

Most airlines allow the stoma products to be in hand luggage. It is wise to ask for an Aisle seat closest to the toilet. It is better to carry all the medicines that are necessary for a trouble free journey especially anti-diarrhea tablets, and rehydration tablets. One must not forget to carry deodorant.

Always empty your pouch in the departure lounge before boarding your flight. It is better to inform the airline staff/cabin crew about your condition and get all the helps from them.

## Eating Tips on Travel

Avoid eating gassy drinks, foods that increase the wind and increases the output like cabbage, onions, eggs and spicy foods. Better to eat lower fiber foods. One should be careful in taking food during travel because there is an increased risk for diarrhea or dehydration. It is better to avoid alcohol during travel.

## Maintaining Secrecy and Confidentiality

It is up to the ostomate to decide who to tell about their ostomy surgery. It is better to inform people closest to you or the loved ones. This will allow you to cope with your emotions and also may ease the fears in your loved ones.

### ■ SEX AND INTIMACY

Some people start thinking about sex immediately after surgery. They may have been unable to participate sexually due to weakness or illness for quite a long-time prior to surgery and are raring to go afterwards. Once again, these patients sometimes are disappointed the first time they attempt to have sex because their bodies have not had enough time to recover.

It is the time to sort through these things and decide if they are really from your surgery and illness or 'ancient history' — the sexual 'baggage' you are carrying around with you. Be honest with yourself and take some time to think about it and discuss things with your partner. Seek professional help from a counselor, your physician, or a sex therapist. Talking really helps.

- Always practice SAFE SEX (foams, lubricated condoms, other forms of contraception).
- Focus on your feelings, not the pouch.
- Empty the pouch before engaging in sexual activity.
- Make sure that the pouch is secure; reinforce it with paper tape around the edges.
- If you wear an ostomy pouch belt, make sure it is clean.
- Make sure you are clean — better yet, jump in the tub or shower together.
- If you are concerned about the appearance of the pouch use a pouch cover or a pouch you cannot see through
- Use a 'passion pouch' during sex. These are smaller, closed-end, disposable pouches that are shorter and less bulky than standard drainable pouches. There are many brands available.
- The 'side-lying' position may work better on the stoma side because the pouch will fall away and not come between you and your partner.
- If you have a colostomy and you irrigate, irrigating just before you have sex might allow you to wear a small patch or 'security pouch' during that time.

### ■ BIBLIOGRAPHY

1. Caring for your Ileostomy and Colostomy
   https://www.mskcc.org/cancer-care/patient-education/caring-for-your-ileostomy-colostomy

2. Feel confident after ostomy surgery-Coplast Canada.
   https://www.coloplast.ca/ostomy/people-with-an-ostomy/after-ostomy-surgery/
3. Intestinal Stomas—Principles, Techniques and Management; second edition, revised and expanded. Edited by Peter A Cataldo, John M Meckaigan; Preoperative considerations-Alang G Thorson.
4. Intimacy with an Ostomy-Convatec.
   https://www.convatec.co.in/ostomy/living-with-an-ostomy/intimacy
5. Psychological attitude to self-appraisal of stoma patients: prospective
   https://thesurgery.or.kr/Synapse/Data/PDFData/6037ASTR/astr-86-152.pdf
6. Role of the enterostomal therapy nurse in ostomy patient rehabilitation.
   https://www.ncbi.nlm.nih.gov/pubmed/1511389
7. United Ostomy Associations of America, Inc. Intimacy after Ostomy Surgery Guide. A publication of the United Ostomy Associations of America, inc. revised 2009. GwenTurnbull, BS, RN, ET, Clearwater, Florida.

# Tips for Maintenance of Stoma

## ■ COLOSTOMY IRRIGATION

Education for the patient with a descending or sigmoid colostomy may include instruction in colostomy irrigation. The appropriateness of routine irrigation as a method of management is initially assessed, and the patient is then counseled regarding management options. The patient who is determined to be a candidate for routine irrigation and elects this management approach is instructed in the procedure.

## ■ CRITERIA FOR IRRIGATION

Patients who meet the following criteria are good candidates for management with routine irrigation:

- *Descending or sigmoid colostomy*: Routine irrigation is a management option only for patients with a descending or sigmoid colostomy. It is an inappropriate approach for patients with a more proximal stoma, because such stomas produce more fluid, higher-volume output; since these patients are unable to regulate fecal output with irrigation, routine irrigation may induce fluid electrolyte imbalance.

> Lukewarm water of 1 to 1.5 liters is advisable for irrigation

- *Normal bowel function*: Routine irrigation is most appropriate for persons with a history of regular, formed bowel movements. This method is least likely to be effective in individuals with frequent episodes of diarrhea or the irregular bowel pattern of irritable colon.
- *Ability to learn and perform the procedure*: Patients must be Capable of learning and performing the irrigation procedure. In addition, they must have access to adequate toilet facilities, such as running water and indoor plumbing.
- *Patient preference*: Irrigation is optional; it is not required to maintain normal bowel function. The decision to use this management approach should be made by the patient, not the healthcare team.

*Some conditions and situations that may be regarded as relative contraindications for routine irrigation include the following:*

- *Stoma prolapse or peristomal hernia*: Because of the potential for increased

> Size of the family, number of toilets, sharing of one toilet by many...in these cases patient may defer irrigation

prolapse or bowel perforation, irrigation should be done only with appropriate equipment.

- *Children and adolescents*: Routine irrigation may not be appropriate for younger patients because of the amount of time required for the procedure and the need to follow a regular schedule.
- *Pelvic or abdominal radiation*: Irrigation is contraindicated in patients who are receiving pelvic or abdominal radiation. It should not be initiated or resumed until the inflammation has resolved, as indicated by restoration of normal bowel function and healthy stomal mucosa.
- *Temporary colostomy*: Routine irrigation is usually not recommended for patients with temporary colostomies because of the time required to master the procedure.
- *Poor prognosis*: Routine irrigation usually is not recommended for patients who have a poor prognosis because of the time and energy required for the procedure. However, candidacy must be determined according to the individual's status and priorities.

## ▨ PRINCIPLES OF COLOSTOMY IRRIGATION (FIGS. 15.1 TO 15.4)

The goal of irrigation is to distend the bowel, making it contract and evacuate its contents. Routine irrigation causes the bowel to empty on a regular basis, which reduces the chance of fecal elimination between irrigations.

1. Irrigation is needed for Colostomy and not for ileostomy
2. During discomfort, distension of abdomen, or when stools get harder- Irrigation works
3. Timing of Irrigation to be customized according to the profession and priorities of the patient

### Scheduling of Irrigation

Most individuals irrigate the colostomy daily or every other day, depending on their preoperative bowel pattern. The time of day is selected on the basis of their individual lifestyles and preferences.

### Type and Volume of Solution

Most patients use lukewarm tap water for irrigation. The alternative is saline, which can be made by adding 2 tsp of salt to 1 quart of water. The volume is titrated for the individual. The goal is to use enough irrigant to distend the colon but not enough to cause cramping pain. Most adults use between 600 and 1000 mL of water. The patient is instructed to instil the irrigant at a steady

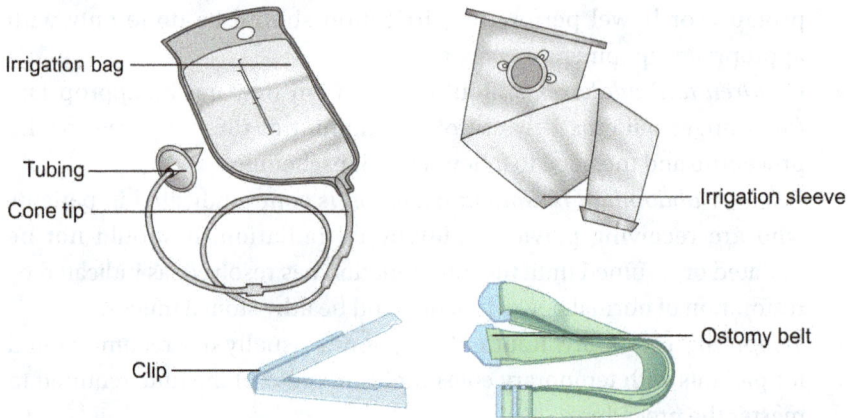

**Fig. 15.1:** Learning of proper irrigation techniques, keeping things ready for irrigation and seeking for a demo from experts would facilitate easy execution of the procedure

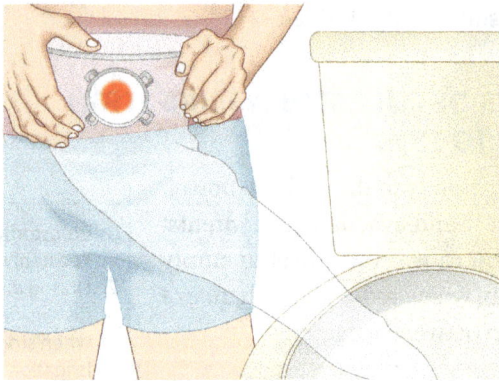

**Fig. 15.2:** One end of the irrigation sleeve attached to the belt with the other end positioned for the direct gushing of irrigation water into the toilet

rate until the feeling of fullness has been achieved. Remind patients who are traveling to use potable water for their irrigations.

## Equipment (Figs. 15.2, 15.3 and 15.5)

A cone tip rather than a catheter is recommended. The cone tip prevents bowel perforation and also acts as a plug to prevent backflow of the irrigating solution around the device. An irrigation sleeve is snapped onto a two piece wafer or belted into place around the stoma. Disposable adhesive irrigation sleeves also may be used. The end of the sleeve can be closed with a clip or placed in the toilet to direct the flow of return.

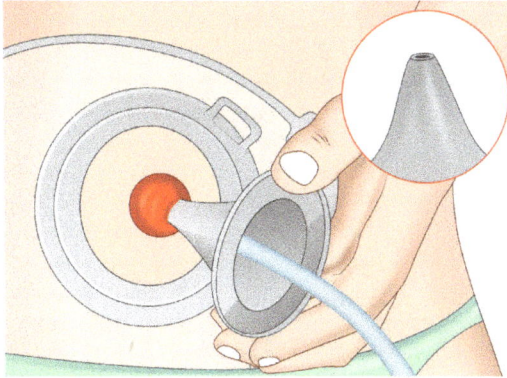

**Fig. 15.3:** For easy insertion of the cone into the stoma, moisten the tip of the cone with a lubricant and gently insert to minimise leakage

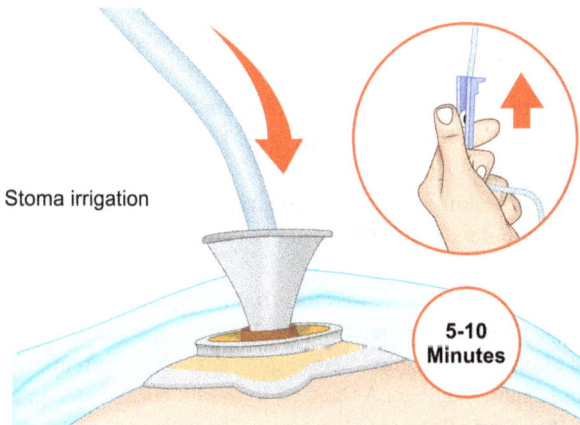

Stoma irrigation

5-10 Minutes

**Fig. 15.4:** Irrigating the stoma. Allowing the water slowly from the irrigation bag into the cone will ensure complete irrigation

## Time Frame

The time frame required for the entire irrigation procedure is usually about 1 hr: approximately 10 min for setup and instillation of irrigant, 30–40 min for evacuation, and 10 min for clean up.

It is not advisable to opt for irrigation during abdominal crams

While waiting for evacuation, the individual is free to pursue other activities with the irrigation sleeve in place.

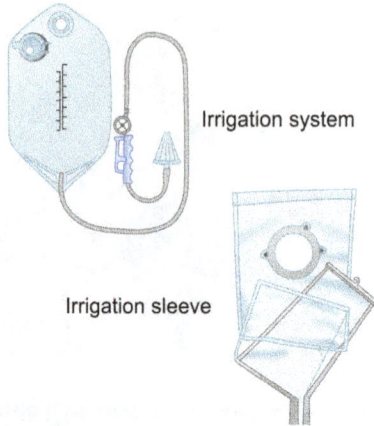

**Fig. 15.5:** Equipments of irrigation. Irrigation system comprises an irrigating container, long tube and a plastic cone shaped device. Irrigation sleeve carries the irrigation ouput into the toilet

## ▪ BIBLIOGRAPHY

1. Colostomy care. www.drugs.com/cg/colostomy-care.html
2. How to apply (change) a colostomy bag? http://www.ostomysoftware.com/OstomyArticles/apply_ostomy_bag.html
3. How to clean the skin around the Stoma? http://www.shieldhealthcare.com/community/popular/2013/02/08/ostomy-care-how-to-clean-the-skin-around-the-stoma/
4. How to deal with your Colostomy bag? http://www.medicinenet.com/colostomy_a_patients_perspective/page5.htm
5. Intestinal Stomas - Principles, Techniques and Management; second edition, revised and expanded; Peter A Cataldo, John M Meckaigan; Stoma Therapy-Ian C. Lavery,Paul Erwin-Toth.
6. Ostomy tips and tricks-Ostomy land-http://www.ostomyland.com/ostomyland/chapter-23-ostomists-top-tips/
7. Pic.courtesy: http://www.wikihow.com/Irrigate-Your-Colostomy

# Patient Related Problems in Stoma

## ▓ INTRODUCTION

A surgeon always tries to construct a good stoma for the well-being of the patient, but then, the stoma that is created is an abnormal opening which takes time to be adapted by the Ostomate physically, mentally and function normally.

Even after creating a good healthy stoma over a period of time, there are several issues and problems which the patient will face during his/her life and these may have different manifestations. It is the duty of the surgeon and the ET nurse to educate the patient.

### Control of Gas and Odor

The two major sources of intestinal gas are swallowed air and gas formed through bacterial action on undigested carbohydrates. Swallowed air is absorbed gradually during its transit throughout the intestinal tract. Therefore, it is more likely to affect the patient with a small bowel stoma especially one located in the proximal small bowel. Since swallowed air is increased by the use of straws, talking while eating, chewing gum, and smoking, the patient who swallows large amounts of air may benefit from reduction or elimination of these practices. Gas formed by bacterial action on undigested carbohydrates is of greater significance to the patient with a large bowel stoma because most Gas-forming foods (e.g. beans, cabbage, broccoli, brussels sprouts, and beer) are identified. The lag time between intake of gas-producing foods and actual flatulence is about 6 hours for the person with a colostomy (based on average transit time from mouth to colon). The individual can decide to omit these foods or to eat them only at times when flatulence will not cause embarrassment. Foods associated with reduced odor include yogurt, parsley, and orange juice. Measures for muffling flatus sounds include applying pressure to the stoma with the hand or elbow. Patients with large amount of flatus but firm stool may benefit from pouches with deodorizing flatus filters. Such filters vent the gas through a charcoal filter, thus eliminating flatus odor while keeping the pouch relatively flat. However, loose stool may seep into the filter, causing odor and leakage.

The most important odor-control measures are the use of odor proof pouches and good hygiene (i.e. keeping the bottom or 'tail' of the pouch clean).

The patient who is using an odor proof pouch and keeps the pouch spout clean should note fecal odor only when the pouch is emptied or changed. It is often helpful to remind the patient that fecal odor during elimination is normal. Additional options for odor control include pouch deodorants, room deodorants, and oral deodorizing agents. Agents used as pouch deodorants include commercial deodorants, commercial perineal cleansers, and mouthwashes, all of which contain antibacterial agents. Deodorizing agents for use in the pouch are added to the pouch after it has been emptied. Room deodorant sprays can be used when the pouch is being emptied or changed. They are particularly beneficial when the patient must empty the pouch in a public restroom, and they are available in purse or pocket size. Oral agents commonly used include Bismuth subgallate (Devrom) and Chlorophyllin copper (Derifil) complex. When taken consistently, these over-the-counter agents reduce fecal odor significantly. Again, it must be emphasized that the best odor-control measures are a secure, odor proof pouch and good hygiene. Oral charcoal capsules are available but may interfere with the absorption of fat-soluble vitamins.

## Management of Diarrhea

The person with a fecal diversion is just as susceptible to episodes of diarrhea as the individual whose bowel is intact. Diarrhea may occur as a result of a viral or bacterial gastroenteritis, antibiotic therapy, radiation therapy, chemotherapy, some medications (e.g. antacids containing magnesium), or food intolerance. Management of diarrhea depends on the location of the stoma within the gastrointestinal tract and the length and function of the proximal bowel. The principles of management are the same for all patients and can be summarized as follows:

- Eliminate the cause of diarrhea if possible; for example, the patient who is taking antibiotics may benefit from a preparation of *Lactobacillus* to restore normal bowel flora.
- Maintain a bland, constipating diet. Recommended foods include rice, pasta, cheese, bananas, and apple sauce.
- Replace fluid and electrolytes. The patient is instructed to replace both fluid volume and fluid components (electrolytes). One approach is to drink a glass of replacement fluid each time the pouch is emptied. Suggested replacement fluids include fruit or vegetable juices and both.
- Over-the-counter anti-diarrheal medications are usually acceptable. One exception is for the patient receiving radiation therapy. Such patients should not take over-the-counter anti-diarrheal agents because many of these preparations contain bismuth which is a metallic agent. Patients should also be instructed to notify their physician of signs and symptoms

of fluid-electrolyte imbalance such as weakness, lethargy, dry mouth and tongue, reduced urine output and increased urine concentration, abdominal cramps, and dizziness when standing. Notifying the physician is particularly important for patients with a small bowel or proximal large bowel stoma because these patients are at increased risk for fluid and electrolyte imbalance during episodes of increased fluid loss.

## Recognition and Management of Food Blockage

Adherence to the guidelines for adding high-fiber foods to the diet usually prevents development of food blockage. The person with an ileostomy however, should be taught the signs and symptoms of food blockage, appropriate home management, and indications for notifying the physician. Signs and symptoms of food blockage are the same as for any intestinal obstruction and vary depending on the degree of obstruction. A partial obstruction usually causes cramping abdominal pain, watery output with a foul odor, and possible abdominal distention and stoma swelling; nausea and vomiting also may occur. With complete obstruction, stoma output ceases; severe cramping pain, abdominal distension, stomal swelling, nausea, and vomiting usually occur. Patients are taught to notify their physician or ET nurse promptly if signs of complete obstruction does not respond to the use of mild analgesics and cessation of eating or drinking. These patients usually require ileal lavage, as outlined in the discussion of obstruction.

## Prevention and Management of Fluid-Electrolyte Imbalance

Persons with an Ileostomy have lost the absorptive functions provided by the colon. They lose approximately 500–750 mL of fluid daily through the stoma compared with 100–200 mL lost by the average person with an intact colon. Thus the individual with an ileostomy is at much greater risk for fluid-electrolyte imbalance when increased loss occurs—for example, with gastroenteritis causing diarrhea and vomiting. Self-care instruction for these patients should focus on the importance of vigorous replacement of fluid and electrolytes during periods of increased loss and on the recognition and prompt response to signs and symptoms of fluid-electrolyte imbalance. The importance of notifying the physician promptly if fluid cannot be replaced during period of increased loss also must be stressed.

## ■ FUNDAMENTALS OF PATIENT CARE

### Special Considerations with Transverse Colostomy

Issues specific to patients with a transverse colostomy include dietary and fluid modifications and concealment of the stoma. Since transverse colostomies most commonly are performed for temporary diversions, an additional issue for many patients is incorporation of the colostomy into their own lifestyle on a temporary basis.

## Dietary and Fluid Modification (Table 16.1)

Nutrients are digested and absorbed in the small intestine. Since the small intestine is not affected by a transverse colostomy, patients with a transverse colostomy have no absolute restrictions imposed by the colostomy. They do lose additional fluid through the stoma and should be instructed to increase fluid intake to 10 glasses of liquid per day.

## Concealment of Stoma

Patients with a transverse colostomy may have a stoma located in the upper abdomen above the belt line. They frequently have concerns related to clothing and concealment of the stoma. Although suggestions must be individualized for the patient, general guidelines include wearing a layer of knit clothing next to the body to keep the pouch secure and smooth and adding a loose outer layer of clothing for concealment. Patients may also find vests, sweaters, scarves, and jackets to be helpful in concealing the stoma.

**Table 16.1:** Trouble managing and troubleshooting foods for ostomates

| Stoma obstructing | Odor producing | Increased/loose stool | Gas-producing |
|---|---|---|---|
| 1. Apple peels | 1. Asparagus | 1. Alcoholic beverage | 1. Alcoholic beverage |
| 2. Raw cabbage | 2. Baked beans | 2. Whole grains | 2. Beans |
| 3. Corn | 3. Broccoli | 3. Bran cereals | 3. Cabbage |
| 4. Coconut | 4. Egg | 4. Cooked cabbage | 4. Cauliflower |
| 5. Dried fruits | 5. Fish | 5. Fresh fruits | 5. Cucumber |
| 6. Mushrooms | 6. Garlic | 6. Milk | 6. Carbonated drinks |
| 7. Orange | 7. Onion | 7. Prunes | 7. Chewing gums |
| 8. Pineapple | 8. Peanut butter | 8. Raisins | 8. Dairy products |
| 9. Nuts | 9. Strong cheese | 9. Spices | 9. Milk/nuts |
| 10. Popcorn | 10. Some vitamins | 10. Apple juice | 10. Onions |
| **Constipation relief** | **Odor control** | **Loose stool control** | **Reducing flatus** |
| 1. Coffee warm/hot | 1. Butter milk | 1. Apple sauce | 1. Cranberry juice |
| 2. Fruits/vegetables cooked | 2. Cranberry juice | 2. Boiled rice | 2. Buttermilk |
| 3. Tomato juice | 3. Water | 3. White bread | 3. Peppermint oil |
| 4. Yoghurt | 4. Mild laxatives | 4. Potato | **Color changes** |
| 5. Peppermint oil | 5. Fresh fruits | 5. Pasta | 1. Food color |
| 6. Fruit juice | | 6. Marshmalows | 2. Iron pills |
| | | | 3. Strawberry |
| | | | 4. Asparagus |
| | | | 5. Beets |
| | | | 6. Tomato sauce |

## Prevention and Management of Constipation

The patient's previous bowel habits—including history of constipation, past management of constipation, and lifestyle factors (e.g. activity level

> Butter, Cheese and Jam could cause constipation

and intake of fiber and fluid affecting bowel function)—must be assessed. It should be explained to the patient that a colostomy does not prevent constipation; specific recommendations must be made for maintenance of healthy bowel function and prevention of constipation. Routine preventive measures include daily exercise and an adequate intake of fluids and fiber. Individual recommendations are made based on usual fluid and fiber intake, past bowel patterns, and activity tolerance. For example, the sedentary patient with a history of constipation and the usual intake of fluid and fiber [limited to 6 glasses of fluid a day and one serving of fiber (<5g)] may be instructed to begin a simple graduated walking program, add 2 glasses of fluid a day, and take a bulk laxative twice daily. An alternative suggestion would be to increase the dietary intake of bulk or to add bran to the diet.

### ■ BIBLIOGRAPHY

1. A handbook for new ostomy patients
   http://www.vcn.bc.ca/ostomyvr/NEW%20PATIENTS%20EDITION%205th%20printing%20web.pdf
2. Colostomy-United Ostomy Association of America Inc.
   http://www.ostomy.org/uploaded/files/ostomy_info/ColostomyNPG_2015s.pdf?direct=1
3. Common stoma problems
   http://www.fittleworth.net/wpsystem/wp-content/uploads/CSP0315-11-fittleworthmedicine.pdf
4. Intestinal Stomas - Principles, Techniques and Management; second edition, revised and expanded; Peter A Cataldo, John M Meckaigan; Stoma Therapy-Ian C Lavery, Paul Erwin-Toth
5. Stoma complications-best practice for clinicians
   http://c.ymcdn.com/sites/www.wocn.org/resource/resmgr/Publications/Stoma_Complications_Best_Pra.pdf

# Educating the Stoma Patient

## ■ TEACHING AND COUNSELING FOR SELF-CARE

The initial focus in patient teaching is on self-care skills and daily management issues, such as dietary alternations. Once these basic skills have been mastered, the focus shifts to how to incorporate the ostomy into the person's lifestyle. With decreasing length of stay in hospital, this is often begun in the hospital and continued at home with a visiting nurse and/or during outpatient visits. Common concerns include bathing and clothing; management of the ostomy at work, during exercise, in recreational activities and travel, and during sexual activity; and disclosure issues.

## ■ BATHING

Patients may take a tub bath or shower with the pouch left on or taken off. They are encouraged to bathe with the pouch on unless it is time to change the pouch (routine bathing with the pouch off may result in inadvertent removal of the skin barrier paste or washing of the skin barrier wafer or ring, which in turn contributes to premature disruption of the pouch seal). The patient may choose to "picture frame" the edges of the pouch with waterproof tape to increase the resistance; the alternative is to pat the taped edges dry or to dry them with a hair dryer on a low setting.

## ■ CLOTHING

Snug undergarments over the pouch help conceal the presence of the stoma. Pouch covers protect the skin from the plastic of the pouch and also serve to conceal the pouch contents. For patients with a flush or slightly protruding stoma located in the lower abdominal quadrants, these measures are usually sufficient to conceal the stoma and allow preoperative clothing to be worn. Clothing modifications usually are minimal for these patients; for example, patients may wear slacks or skirts that have front pleats or are loose-fitting. Women are instructed that pantyhose and stretch panty girdles are permissible. Regular girdles may also be worn provided that the stays do not cross the stoma. Bathing suits are available that effectively conceal the stoma; women are advised to look for patterned suits with shirring or draping. Patients should also be made aware of specialty underclothing designed for the person with an ostomy.

# ■ FECAL DIVERSIONS

When the distal bowel segment remains intact—as with a loop stoma, a double-barrel stoma, or an end stoma with Hartmann's pouch—the patient must be prepared for temporary output of stool per rectum once peristalsis returns. The distal bowel continues to produce mucus, and the patient may periodically feel rectal fullness and the need to evacuate the accumulated mucus. Patients who sense rectal distention but are unable to expel the mucus may benefit from a low-volume rectal enema to flush out the mucus. The patient who has a double-barrel ostomy must be taught how to manage the nonfunctioning "mucous fistula" stoma. If the distal mucous fistula stoma is immediately adjacent to the proximal functioning stoma, it should be included in the pouch. If the nonfunctioning stoma is located at a distance from the proximal stoma, it can be managed with a light dressing, changed by the patient either daily or as needed, or with a stoma cap or cover.

# ■ DISCHARGE PLANNING

Discharge planning is critical for the patient with an ostomy. As the length of stay after ostomy surgery has shortened, the time available for teaching and counseling has also decreased. The teaching focus during the postoperative phase must be survival skills—that is, pouch emptying and pouch changing procedures. Much additional teaching and counseling are required to support integration of the ostomy into the patient's lifestyle. All patients should have access to outpatient follow-up on a regular basis. In addition to such follow-up, many patients need home health care after discharge. The home care nurse can provide reinforcement and support for self-care and additional instruction regarding ostomy management and counseling regarding psychosocial issues. The ET nurse who provides instruction should evaluate the ostomy patient's potential need for home care follow up and should initiate or contribute to the referral. It is frequently beneficial to contact the home care nurse and provide that professional with additional information regarding the patient's care.

# ■ OSTOMATE BILL OF RIGHTS*

1. Be given pre-op counseling
2. Have an appropriately positioned stoma site
3. Have a well-constructed stoma
4. Have skilled postoperative nursing care
5. Have emotional support
6. Have individual instruction
7. Be informed on the availability of supplies

8. Be provided with information on community resources
9. Have post-hospital follow up and life-long supervision
10. Benefit from team efforts of health care professionals
11. Be provided with information and counsel from the ostomy association and its members

*Adopted by the United Ostomy Association House of Delegates at the UOA Annual Conference 1977

## ■ BIBLIOGRAPHY

1. Berman A, Snyder SJ, Kozier B, Erb G. Kozier & Erb's Fundamentals of Nursing: Concepts, Process, and Practice, 8th edn. Upper Saddle River, NJ: Pearson Education, Inc. 2008. pp. 1345-9.
2. Burke KM, LeMone P, Mohn-Brown EL, Eby L. Medical-Surgical Nursing Care, 2nd edn. Upper Saddle River, NJ: Pearson Prentice Hall. 2007. pp.457-60, 778-81.
3. Ignatavicius DD, Workman ML. Medical-Surgical Nursing: Patient-Centered Collaborative care, 6th edn. St. Louis, MO: Saunders Elsevier. 2010. pp. 1298-1302, 1325-9, 1576-8.
4. Intestinal Stomas - Principles, Techniques and Management; second edition, revised and expanded; Peter.A. Cataldo, John .M. Meckaigan; Stoma Therapy-Ian C.Lavery,Paul Erwin-Toth.
5. Potter PA, Perry AG. Fundamentals of Nursing, 7th edn. St. Louis, MO: Elsevier Mosby. 2009. pp. 1134, 1210-5.
6. The basics of teaching patients Ostomy care.
   http://www.woundsource.com/blog/basics-teaching-patients-ostomy-care.

# Complications of Stoma

## ■ INTRODUCTION

The complications of stoma are seen with a wide spectrum of problems to the ostomates. The reported overall complication rates vary considerably ranging from 10% to 50%.

There are several factors which are related to the incidence of complications, for example, patients operated in the emergency will have a higher incidence of complication because they may not have had adequate preoperative preparations.

Defunctioning stomas or temporary stomas are associated with lesser complications as compared to the permanent stomas.

## ■ COMPLICATIONS (FLOWCHART 18.1)

The type of complications also depends upon the types of stoma. Ileostomies are associated with higher incidence of skin complications and leakage, while colostomies are associated with higher incidence of odor, prolapse and parastomal hernia. When end stomas are compared with the loop stomas, there seems to be a higher complication with loop stomas.

It is expected that stomas constructed by surgeons with less experience are likely to have more complications, however, this is not been shown in the studies.

The nature of suture material used for creating the stoma has also been implicated in creating complications. For example, monofilament absorbable sutures cause less complication as compared with the braided sutures.

**Flowchart 18.1:** Complications of Stoma according to locations in the GI tract

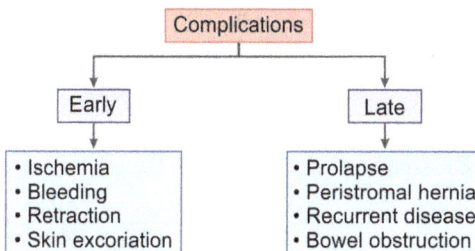

```
                    Complications
                   /            \
              Early              Late
                |                 |
      • Ischemia          • Prolapse
      • Bleeding          • Peristromal hernia
      • Retraction        • Recurrent disease
      • Skin excoriation  • Bowel obstruction
```

There are also other risk factors which may cause complications following a stoma creation. These include:

- Age
- Obesity
- Comorbid condition such as diabetes
- Chronic obstructive pulmonary disease (COPD)
- Preoperative use of steroids
- Lack of preoperative planning
- Crohn's disease
- Smoking, etc.

The complications can be divided into those occurring early or late or according to location in the gastrointestinal (GI) tract (*see* Flowchart 18.1).

Immediate complications are: Necrosis, bowel ischemia, odema, bleeding and hematoma.

Early complications are: Retraction, mucocutaneous seperation, stenosis and peristomal skin irritation, peristomal abscess, fistula, obstruction, wrong limb maturation, wrong site.

Late complications are: Retraction, prolapse, stenosis, obstruction, parastomal hernia, peristomal abscess, fistula, reoccurrence of disease, cancer.

Some of the complications could occur at any time and include diarrhea, constipation, high output stoma and psychosocial problems (Table 18.1). Early post operative complications lead to prolonged hospital stay and increase in costs. Early complications can be caused by the selection of the wrong site, inadequate mobilization, vascular compromise or inadequate pouting.

Late complications could be either a sequel of the early complications, related to the underlying diseases or as a result of the process of healing and fibrosis.

**Table 18.1:** Stomal complications and causes

| Skin problems | Possible causes |
|---|---|
| • Poor stoma sitting | • Allergic skin reactions |
| • Perspiration | • Dressings, etc. |
| • Skin preparation - soaps, etc. | • Psoriasis/eczema |
| • Drug excretion | • Radiotherapy |
| • Drug interactions | • Poor technique |
| • Changes in skin permeability | • Poor hygiene |
| | • Poor general health |

## STOMAL NECROSIS (FIG. 18.1)

It is one of the most serious early complications and its incidence ranges from 0.3% to 20 %.

Ischemia could be mucosal, muscular or full thickness.

Mucosal ischemia generally resolves without sequel.

Submucosa and muscular ischemia leads to fibrosis and stricture formation, while full thickness ischemia is associated with necrosis and perforation.

It is usually more common with colostomy than ileostomy. The ischemia is attributed due to reduced arterial supply or excessive nervous congestion which can compromise bowel perfusion which may lead to necrosis of stoma.

This is a preventable complication if the surgeon maintains the vascularity of the bowel during surgery.

## RETRACTION

When the stoma disappears or protrudes below the skin surface it is called retracted stoma (Fig. 18.2). It is generally recommended both colostomies and ileostomies should be constructed to protrude above the skin surface with ileostommies atleast 2 cm and colostomies atleast 1 cm from the skin surface.

The incidence of stoma retraction ranges from 1% to 32%. A retracted stoma can occur early or late. Usual causes are tension at the mesentry due

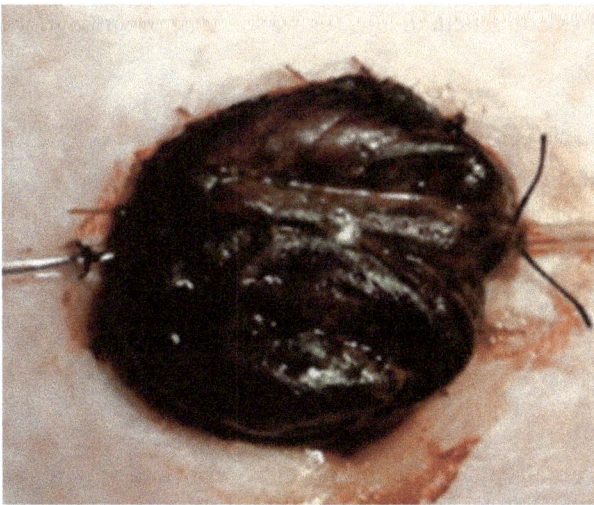

**Fig. 18.1:** Stomal necrosis

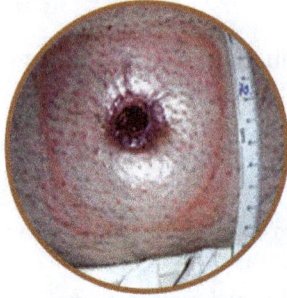

A retracted stoma lies below skin level commonly caused by too short a section of intestine used.
**Management:**
If excess weight/obesity is the case, weight loss should be encouraged. Irrigation if it is a colostomy. Further surgical procedure may be necessary.

**Fig. 18.2:** Retracted stoma

to inadequate mobilization, shortened mesentry, recurrent malignancy, radiation, edema and distention of the bowel, adhesions and scaring in the mesentry, obesity, steroids.

The stoma should be evaluated with the patient sitting and standing to determine the degree of retraction.

## Mucocutaneous Separation

Mucocutaneous separation is the separation of the stoma from the skin at the junction of the skin and intestine used to create stoma. The incidence varies from 3.9% to 25%. It occurs in the early postoperative period and the usual causes include poor wound healing due to malnutrition, steroid therapy, superficial infection, diabetes mellitus, chemotherapy, prior radiation therapy to the abdominal area.

Sometimes a mucocutaneous separation may progress to the retraction of the stoma.

## PERISTOMAL SKIN IRRITATION (FIGS. 18.3 AND 18.4)

This complication can occur at any time following a stoma.

The clinical presentation varies widely from mild peristomal skin irritation to severe excoriation, to ulceration and necrosis.

The triggering factors could be chemical dermatitis caused by the stoma effluent, improper application of a pouch, allergy to any of the components of pouching system such as adhesive, paste, tape, etc.

## Prevention

Prevention entails the selection of an appropriate stoma site, ensuring adequate height of the stoma, attention to fitting of the appliance, regular change of the appliance.

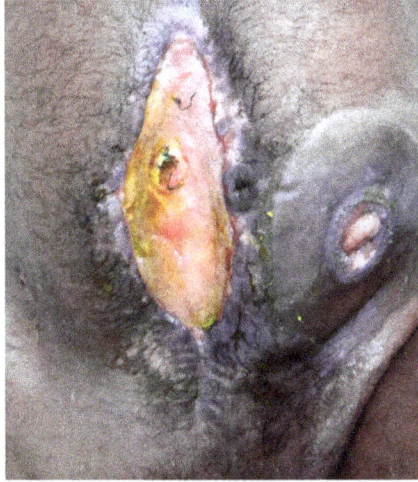

**Fig. 18.3:** Nonfunctioning Colostomy with functioning ileostomy showing Peristomal Granuloma

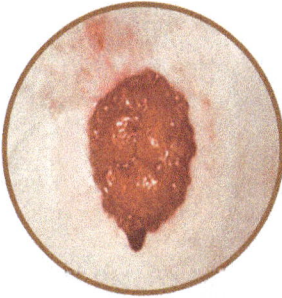

**Granulomas**
Granulomas at the mucosa are seen in the transition between the stoma and the skin causes include chemical or mechanical irritation, it can be treated by covering raised areas with silver nitrate, diathermy (electrical heating), laser treatment.

**Fig. 18.4:** Granulomas

## Metabolic Problems

The normal output from an ileostomy is approximately 800 mL/day. In the immediate postoperative period, the volume may be much higher because of partial obstruction caused by edema of the stoma. In the established stoma a bacterial or viral gastroenteritis commonly increases the output and may require intravenous fluid replacement until the volume of output diminishes. Chronic losses of electrolytes may alter the ratio of chemicals and predispose the patient to the precipitation of stones in the kidneys and gallbladder .If resection of an appreciable length of distal ileum has occurred, the possibility of a vitamin B12 deficiency must be considered. Necrosis occurs because the terminal portion of the bowel has been deprived of an adequate blood supply.

## ■ PARASTOMAL ABSCESS, ULCER, AND FISTULA

They are unusual complications occuring with the frequency of 1% to 3%. It can occur in the immediate postoperative period as a result of skin and soft tissue infection. It can also occur due to infected suture, granuloma, infection of a hematoma at the mucocutaneous junction or due to disease recurrence, (for example, Crohn's disease) or sometimes due to erosion caused by the mesh placed for parastomal hernia

In the early postoperative period, considering the local environment, parastomal abscesses are uncommon. When they do occur, they are related to revision or reconstruction of a stoma at the same site. An abscess which is the result of an infected hematoma or a misplaced suture during maturation, requires surgical drainage. When an abscess develops at a mature stoma, it is usually the result of folliculitis or recurrent Crohn's disease in an ileostomy (Table 18.2).

**Table 18.2:** Showing the possible conditions and causes of Stomal skin complications and their management

| Condition | Cause | Solution |
|---|---|---|
| Allergic | Sensitivity to skin barriers, adhesives, tapes | Use patch test to determine what patient can tolerate |
| Bacterial | Folliculitis | Trim peristomal hair with scissors or electric razor. Use adhesive remover to ease release of adhesives |
| Fungal | *Candida albicans* | Nystatin topical powder is applied with each pouch change. Excess powder must be dusted off to allow appliance to seal |
| Chemical | Leakage of effluent under pouching system | Determine cause of leakage. Check for peristomal fistula. Refit into proper pouching system. Dust skin with skin barrier power prior to pouching. Severe hyperplasia may require surgical debridement and use of nonadherent system until re-epithelialization occurs |
| Mechanical | Skin stripping from adhesive removal. Laceration of stoma from pouching system is due to shifting, improper sizing, or improper application | Gently pull skin away from adhesive with warm, moist gauze square or adhesive remover. Remeasure stoma. Observe pouching system while patient is sitting, supine, and standing. Observe patient applying pouching. |
| Other peristomal abscess | Commonly caused by recurrent Crohn's disease | Unroof ulcer: If ulcer is < 2 cm, cover with nonadherent gauze or hydrocolloid, apply pouch as usual, and change every 2–3 days. If ulcer is > 2 cm, apply nonadherent pouching system. |

At a colostomy, an abscess usually results from perforation of the intestine with an enema tip during attempted irrigation. A parastomal abscess must be drained if it has not drained spontaneously. An ileoscopy or stoma injection is performed to investigate the cause of the abscess and to determine whether a fistula is present. If no fistula is present, the cause is invariably folliculitis. The abscess may be drained, but it will not heal unless the cavity is unroofed by excising the undermined skin.

Re-epithelization then will occur. If the unroofed area is small, the ulcer is managed with a small piece of nonadhesive dressing placed under the conventional ostomy management system and changed daily until it heals.

The dressing used is an absorbent paper pad moistened with aluminum acetate solution. After an abscess has been drained whether or not a fistula is present will become evident. Enteric content will be seen issuing from the drain site or under the ostomy management system and will create skin excoriation. A fistula in an ileostomy is invariably the result of prestomal Crohn's disease. Treatment requires resection of the prestomal disease and construction of a new stoma. It is preferable to relocate the stoma if a suitable site exists so as to avoid the infection present at the old site. This problem is the reason that a midline abdominal incision is advised in surgery for inflammatory bowel disease. A midline incision preserves all quadrants of the abdomen in the event that relocation of a stoma becomes necessary.

A parastomal abscess resulting from a perforated colon is a more serious and urgent problem since the perforation and abscess are usually within the parastomal hernia that precipitated the injury. This situation involves the potential for contamination of the peritoneal cavity. The abscess must be drained and laparotomy must be performed to resect the perforation. If possible, the stoma is relocated and the hernia repaired. This procedure may be staged depending on the patient's toxicity. Pyoderma gangrenosum around a stoma may mimic a parastomal ulcer. This condition is best managed locally with the Perry ostomy management system and conventional medical treatment of the pyoderma. Treatment consists of local applications of a 10–20% solution of benzoyl peroxide which kills bacteria and fungus. A high dose of Tetracycline (100–200 g/day) is given orally. In some instances Dapsone and Colchicine are used. Since Dapsone may produce anemia, the initial dose is 25 mg, and this dose is increased to 100 mg over several months. In addition, patients should be given vitamin E which has a beneficial effect on erythrocytes. Methotrexate or Azathioprine and antibiotics can be used sparingly, and Corticosteroids can be used systemically.

## ▪ PARASTOMAL HERNIA (FIGS. 18.5 AND 18.6)

Parastomal hernia are relatively uncommon with ileostomy; the reported incidence varies between 0.7 and 2.6%. These hernias are more common

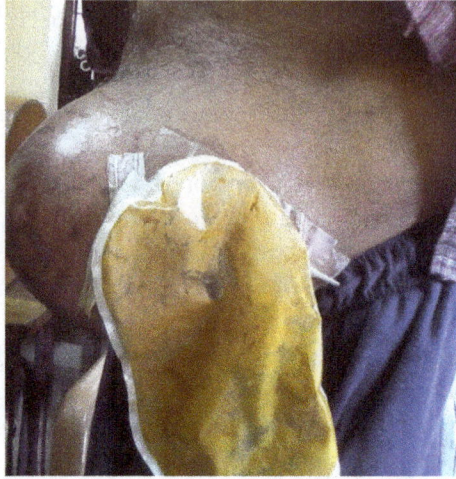

**Fig. 18.5:** Parastomal hernia

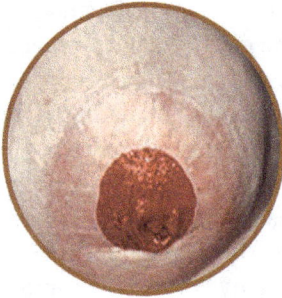

**Hernia**
A bulge around the stoma can
be a true, sliding of 'false' hernia.
True hernia–a loop of the intestine moves through
the hole in the abdominal wall sliding hernia–
a segment of the intestine used to create the stoma
becomes looped into the subcutaneous fatty tissue.
'False' hernia–increased abdominal pressure
produces a bulge in the side of the body due to a
weakened abdominal wall–this is the most common cause.

**Fig. 18.6:** Hernia

with colostomies with occurrences reported as between 3 and 10% of patients. Predisposing conditions are obesity, a large abdominal wall aperture, placement of the stoma lateral to the rectus sheath, and weakness of the abdominal wall from age or multiple incisions. Parastomal hernias is common in peristomal skin conditions cause solution allergic sensitivity to skin barriers. Use patch test to determine adhesives, tapes what patient can tolerate. Trim peristomal hair with scissors or electric razor. Use adhesive remover to ease release of adhesives.

Fungal Candida albicans, Nystatin topical powder is applied with each pouch change.

Excess powder must be dusted off to allow appliance to seal. Chemical leakage of effluent under. Determines cause of leakage, pouching system. Check for peristomal fistula.

Refit into proper pouching system.

Dust skin with skin barrier powder prior to pouching.

Severe hyperplasia may require surgical debridement and use of nonadherent system until re-epithelialization occurs. For shifting, improper sizing, remeasure the stoma. For proper application observe pouching system while patient is sitting, supine, and standing. Observe patient applying pouching.

Other peristomal problems commonly caused by ulcer-Unroof ulcer and abscess. If ulcer is < 2 cm, cover with nonadherent gauze or hydrocolloid, apply pouch as usual, and change every 2-3 days. If ulcer is > 2 cm, apply non adherent gauze.

Pouching system generally enlarge and may cause an unsightly bulge under clothing. If untreated, these hernias may enlarge and make it difficult to keep an ostomy management system attached. If a rigid face plate is used, pressure necrosis may result from tightening the belt to keep the system attached. Less rigid ostomy management systems such as those with a pectin-based skin barrier, make this complication less likely. Smaller, asymptomatic hernias can be managed by using a Velcro binding with an opening cut for the pouching system. The indications for surgery are difficulty with pouch application or with irrigation of the colostomy. Surgery is most satisfactorily done by relocating the stoma usually to the contralateral side. As a practical consideration, certain sites for relocating the stoma are less than optimal, and local repair may be preferable. Local repair is done at laparotomy. The orifice through the abdominal wall is closed with interrupted nonabsorbable sutures. In a survey of patients at the Cleveland Clinic, the cumulative probability of recurrence was 46% after 6 years. Obesity was the only clinical factor investigated that significantly predisposed patient to recurrence of the hernia.

## ■ STRICTURE

It is the narrowing or constriction of the stomal lumen at the level of skin or fascia. The incidence ranges from 2% to 8.7%. It is usually a late complication. It can occasionally occur in the early postoperative period. Sometimes it is due to disease recurrence in patients with Crohn's or malignancy or Ischemic Bowel Disease (IBD).

It is still thought by some individuals that stomas need to be dilated after construction to prevent stricture formation. This idea originated when stomas were not matured primarily.

Patients usually present with change in bowel habits with small caliber of stool, abdominal cramps, explosive diarrhea and increased passage of flatus (Fig. 18.7).

A gentle peristomal examination with a lubricated gloved finger can reveal the sight of stenosis. A novel method for treating mild stenosis is with

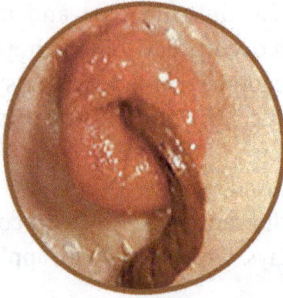

**Stenosis**
The stoma is edematous, mushroom shaped and glistening feces is expelled in the form of a thin strip; the blockage is due to tightened tissue around the stoma can be treated by dilation of the intestine. If at skin level, local surgery may be necessary.

**Fig. 18.7:** Stenosis

the use of stomal plugs. Other methods like insertion of self expanding metal stents, creation of a new stoma has been described at few centers

When stomas are constructed correctly and matured primarily, there is no reason for 'dilatation' of the stoma. This practice is not only uncomfortable and unnecessary but can also cause strictures from the scarring that develops as a result of the repeated trauma caused by the dilatation. If a stricture develops as a result of ischemia or recurrent prestomal Crohn's disease, revision is necessary. Such revision may be done locally, but recurrent Crohn's disease usually requires laparotomy and resection of the terminal ileum.

## ■ CAPUT MEDUSA (FIG. 18.8)

Caput medusa are a circumferential burgundy halo around a stoma that blanches with pressure. It is the result of a portosystemic collateral circulation from portal hypertension. The underlying cause is cirrhosis caused by sclerosing cholangitis. Bleeding, the resulting complication occurs at the mucocutaneous junction and may be profuse. Immediate control of the bleeding can be obtained by applying pressure precisely to the bleeding point. The bleeding will stop if there is no coagulopathy as may occur with cirrhosis. Repeated episodes of bleeding should prompt surgical treatment. Such treatment involves interrupting the portosystemic circulation by separating the mucocutaneous junction. The collateral circulation is located at this level. It is not necessary to mobilize the stoma completely down into the peritoneal cavity. Some of the vessels to be interrupted have a large caliber and require individual ligation. Blood loss may be more than expected, if the portal pressure is high. Because of the pathophysiology of the caput medusae, recurrence is inevitable. Portosystemic shunting surgically or via transjugular intrahepatic portosystemic shunt (TIPS) may be indicated. Sclerotherapy has been proposed as a treatment method, but those reported cases in which it was done required multiple injections and the effect was short-lived.

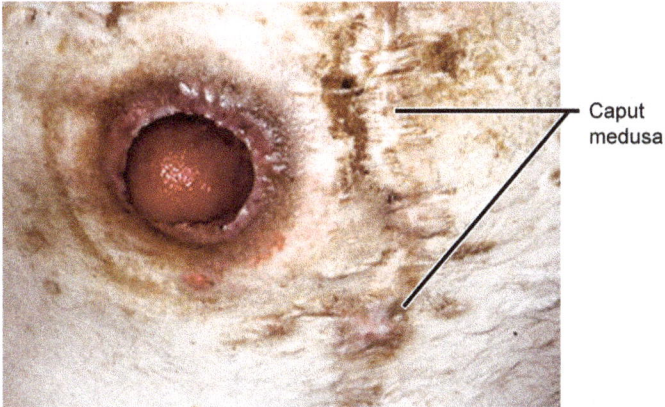

**Fig. 18.8:** Caput medusa

## Obstruction (Fig. 18.9)

This can occur in the early and late postoperative periods. The causes include postoperative adhesion, internal herniation, recurrence of the disease in the form of strictures or disseminated malignancy, stenosis of stoma, complicated parastomal hernia and lastly by a food bolus.

The incidence of obstruction varies from 2.7% to 23%.

In the early postoperative period, obstruction is caused by edema at the level of the new stoma. The obstruction may result in some abdominal cramping and liquid output caused by the excessive secretion of succus entericus. As the time from operation increases and the edema settles, so do the symptoms. In a well-established ileostomy, an adhesive bowel obstruction may occur (as after any abdominal operation). In specific relation to the stoma, obstruction caused by a food bolus needs to be considered. Direct questioning of the patient regarding recent ingestion of food with a high fiber content will given an indication of the probability of such obstruction. If the patient has been indiscreet and has eaten a large volume of high-fiber foods, it is likely that a bolus of undigested food is the cause of the obstruction, the point of obstruction occurs at the fascia level of the abdominal wall. Management involves ileostomy lavage. The lavage is performed by inserting a 22 or 24F. Foley catheter into the distal bowel and irrigating it with several 100-mL aliquots of saline. A two-piece pouching system or irrigation sleeve can be applied to manage the flow. If the catheter can be inserted into the stoma for several inches and irrigation with several aliquots does not produce a return of fluid containing particulate matter of undigested food, the obstruction should be considered more proximal probably an adhesive bowel obstruction. Further attempts to relieve the obstruction by irrigation should be stopped. If the irrigation produces a volume of undigested fibrous

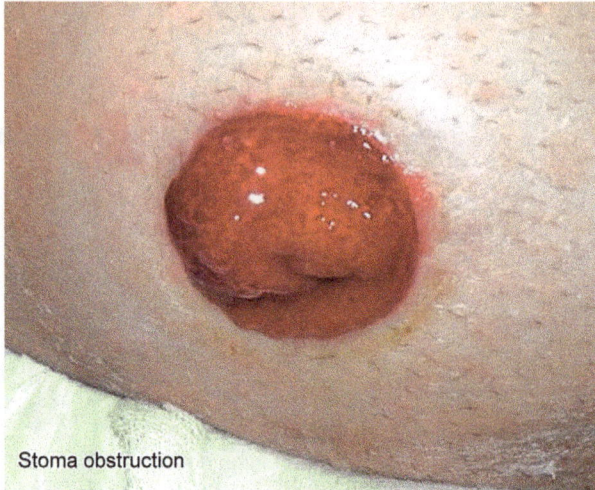

Stoma obstruction

**Fig. 18.9:** Stoma obstruction

material, the procedure is continued until the bolus is broken up and there is some evidence of spontaneous evacuation. Treatment of a bolus obstruction by lavage usually does not require admission to the hospital.

## MUCOSAL IMPLANTS

Mucosal implants are the islands of mucosa that have lodged along suture tracts; they are avoided by using appropriate technique during stoma construction. During maturation of the stoma, the mucocutaneous sutures are placed through the dermal layers of the skin without entering the epidermis. If mucosal implants create a problem, it is from the mucus that they secrete under the ostomy management system. The mucus reduces the adhesion of the pouch and causes leakage. It is not common for implants to cause a major problem, but if the implants are extensive, relocation of the stoma may be necessary. Precise destruction at skin level with a needle electrocautery will give temporary relief.

## STOMAL PROLAPSE (FIG. 18.10)

It refers to the full thickness protrusion of the bowel through the fascial defect. Various contributory factors include redundance of the bowel brought out as stoma, lack of fixation of the bowel, lack of fascial support, wrong position, large opening, obesity, poor muscle tone, increased intra-abdominal pressure and pregnancy.

The overall incidence varies from 2% to 25%. There are two types of stomal prolapse - fixed and sliding. In the fixed prolapse, the fixed length of

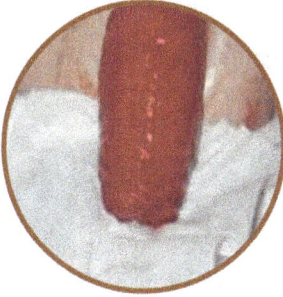

The section of intestine used to create the colostomy is almost turned inside out and pushed forward it can be treated by gently pushing the prolapsed segment back into the abdomen if oedematous, use ice to reduce blood flow and sugar to reduce the edema

**Fig. 18.10:** Stomal prolapse

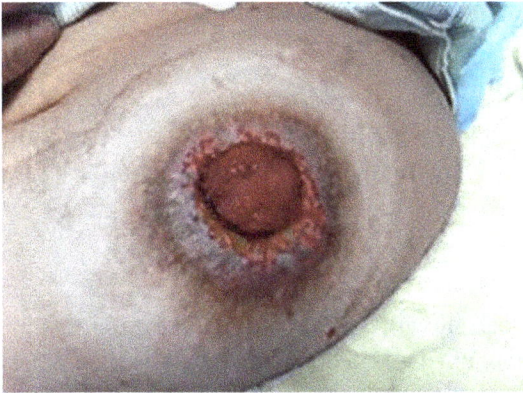

**Fig. 18.11:** Peristomal varices

the bowel prolapses, whereas in the sliding prolapse, the bowel prolapses whereever there is an increase in the intra-abdominal pressure.

Though most patients are asymptomatic, the condition is alarming and mentally distressing for the patient and their relatives.

### ■ BLEEDING AND PERISTOMAL VARICES (FIG. 18.11)

Bleeding is one of the common early postoperative complications. It is due to inadequate hemostasis, trauma to the mucosal surface or coagulopathy. In the late phase, it can be due to excessive granulation tissue formation around the stoma, varices, trauma to stoma due to ill fitting appliances, recurrence of disease and malignancy.

Peristomal varices are seen in patients with portal hypertension. It is seen at the juntion of stoma with the skin. These are vulnerable to bleed with minor trauma. It is a rare complication which can also occur following ileostomy done in the setting of ulcerative colitis with primary scelerosing colangitis.

## ■ RECURRENCE OF DISEASE

Malignancy and inflammatory bowel disease can occur at the site of stoma. Any complaints of bleeding, pain, obstruction, growth should be evaluated and treated accordingly.

## ■ DIVERSION COLITIS

This is seen in patients with end ileostomy or end colostomy. Segments of large intestine that are diverted away from the fecal flow are affected. It is due to the deficiency of short chain fatty acids (SCFAs) and other luminal nutrients in colonocytes. Most of the patients remain asymptomatic and the findings are seen on endoscopy. Sometimes they present with bleeding per rectum, abdominal pain and mucous discharge.

## ■ DIARRHOEA

Stomal diarrhoea is similar to diarrhea in normal patients. It is managed conservatively with oral rehydration and dietary modifications. But it is often self remedy.

## ■ CONSTIPATION

This is seen exclusively with the colostomy. The causes are similar to a normal person. Treatment involves encouraging oral fluids, high fiber diet and usage of laxatives.

## ■ PARTIAL OR INCOMPLETE DIVERSION

This is often done to protect a distal anastamosis. But at times the diversion may be incomplete leading to passage of some fecal matter into the distal limb. If the anastomosis has not healed it can lead to anastomotic leak and pelvic sepsis.

It has been reported that 15% of loop colostomies diverted the fecal stream incompletely from as early as 3rd postoperative month. This is due to retraction of the distal limb.

## ■ TRAUMA

Trauma to the stoma may occur in body contact sports, but this is uncommon because most patients with stomas avoid this type of activity. When the aperture in the pouching system is too small or misplaced, vigorous physical activity may result in a cut or a circumferential ulcer and bleeding. If the cut is most common, reasons for stoma revision are technical errors and recurrent disease. Surgeons, in concern with ET nurses, must approach the construction of stomas with care and make every effort to minimize potential problems, both physical and psychosocial.

## ■ TIPS FOR PREVENTION, EARLY DEDUCTION AND MANAGEMENT OF SIMPLE COMPLICATIONS

- The stoma should be carefully examined in the early postoperative period to detect complications early.
- The normal mucosa is rose to brick red in color. Pallor may indicate anemia. Blanching, dark red or purple color indicates inadequate blood supply to the stoma.
- Blackish discoloration indicates necrosis.
- The stoma should be assessed and color documented every 8 hours. There should be mild to moderate edema in the first 5 to 7 postoperative days.
- Severe edema may indicate obstruction of the stoma. Initially the stoma may ooze on touch.
- For the colostomy patient, there are essentially no food restrictions but for the ileostomy patient it is important to avoid some food to prevent intestinal blockage.
- Patients should be encouraged to eat at regular intervals, chew food well and drink adequate fluids.
- Fecal output can be 1,000 to 1,500 mL every 24 hours.
- Enteric coated, time released capsules or hard tablets may not be absorbed by the patient who has had an ileostomy. Liquid or chewable medicines are preferred.
- Patients need vitamins A, D, E and K supplemented since colon absorption and synthesis are eliminated.
- In case of a food block, the patient should be placed in the knee-chest position and the area below the stoma should be massaged gently.
- Bad odor can have a major impact on quality of life. Built in charcoal filters can be used.
- A cup of tea is a patient's best friend (antispasmodic). Walking is nature's tranquilizer.
- Routine skin care: The pouch should be gently pulled away from the skin while supporting the skin. Avoid wiping the area with paper towels or toilet paper that leave a lot of fibers behind.
- If the peristomal skin is hairy it should be shaved regularly to prevent folliculitis and pain during removal of the pouch.
- Patients should be cautioned not to lift anything over 5 kg for the first 6 to 8 weeks after surgery.
- Pregnancy and child birth are possible normally but it is better to have a prior consultation with the treating physician.

- Before the patient is discharged they should be able to demonstrate cleaning and changing the pouch, know where to obtain supplies, know how to contact resource person for problem and know how/when to follow-up with the physician, ostomy staff and support group if available.
- The opening of the flange should be about 1/8 inch larger than the stoma. The pouch should be emptied when it is no more than 1/3 full and to cleanse the pouch from the bottom with the squeeze bottle filled with water.
- Colostomy irrigation is a good method to establish regularity and relieve constipation. Patients who are to be started on colostomy irrigation are assessed for past bowel habits and frequency of stools, location of colostomy, age, independence, dexterity, general health and personal preferance.

## ■ BIBLIOGRAPHY

1. Carlstedt A, Fasth S, Hulten L, et al. Long-term ileostomy complications in patients with ulcerative colitis and Crohn's disease. Int J Colorectal Dis. 1987;2(1):22-25.
2. Green EW. Colostomies and their complications. Surg Gynecol Obstet. 1966; 122(6):1230-2.
3. Goligher JC, Herbert Livingstone, Duthie Herold, Nixon Homewood. Surgery of the Anus, Rectum and Colon. 5th ed. London: Bailliere Tindall; 1984.
4. Intestinal Stomas by Peter A Cataldo, John M Meckaigan. Stoma Therapy Ian C. Lavery and Paul Erwin-Toth The Cleveland Clinic Foundation, Cleveland, Ohio, USA pp. 81-8.
5. McLeod RS, Lavery IC, Leatherman JR, et al. Factors affecting quality of life with conventional ileostomy. World J Surg. 1986;10(3):474-80.
6. Prian GW, Sawyer RB, Sawyer, KC. Repair of peristomal colostomy hernias. Am J Surg. 1975;130(6):694-6.

# Teaching Ostomy Care to Nursing Students

## ▣ INTRODUCTION

Every year more than a lakh people in India undergo ostomy surgery with the creation of GI or urinary stoma. Many others have temporary ostomies. The number of Ostomates in India cannot be cared individually by enterostomal therapy (ET) nurses. This is because of the dearth of ET nurses, non-availability of ET nurses in the cities other than Metros. This situation is still compounded to the illiterates, poor and patients without family support.

There are also patients who are not aware of such facilities and also their relatives who are at difficulty in obtaining stoma care facility and its products. Hence it is better if student nurses are taught about ostomy care in their curriculum by a qualified ET nurse.

## ▣ PLANNING AND TEACHING OF OSTOMY TO STUDENT NURSES

Students require knowledge about concepts and a variety of principles to enable them to care for a patient with an ostomy.

Student nurses need to acquire a positive attitude about ostomy. Before beginning to care for patients with ostomies, students often express both fear and disgust at the prospect of dealing and coping with ostomies.

Because of their own feelings they may not notice the individual behind the stoma. These feelings can be addressed by use of a group process. Having an ET nurse as an facilitator in the group process is often helpful. Hence a student nurse would need to learn about the development of body image after creation of stoma.

Students' nurses must be equipped with the knowledge of the normal Anatomy and Physiology of the GI system and urinary systems and alterations in them. They then require knowledge about types of stomas, normal functioning of stomas, skin care, the mechanics of applying the pouching systems and how to effectively utilize an ET nurse as a consultant.

In a nut shell, the ET nurses' collaboration with the school of nursing ensures that student nurses and new graduates will have the correct and current information about the care of the patient with stoma.

# ■ BIBLIOGRAPHY

1. Doughty D. Principles of ostomy management in the oncology patient. J Support Oncol. 2005;3(1):59-69.
2. Fulham J. Providing dietary advice for the individual with a stoma. Br J Nurs. 2008;17(2):522-7.
3. IA BPG-International affairs and best practice guidelines -Transforming nursing through practice-clinical best practice guidelines,Aug2009 Ostomy care and Management. http://rnao.ca/sites/rnao-ca/files/Ostomy_Care__Management.pdf
4. Mullen BD, McGinn KA. The Ostomy Book: Living Comfortably with Colostomies, Ileostomies, and Urostomies, 3rd edn. Boulder, CO: Bull Publishing Co; 2008.

# Role of Ostomy Visitor

## ■ INTRODUCTION

*"The well being of the ostomate is the ultimate goal of the partnership between the surgeon, the stoma nurse and the trained ostomy visitor."*

Ostomy visitor is defined as a person who has undergone ostomy surgery and is now leading a normal life. His or her purpose is to visit the patient who is about to go for ostomy or has undergone one to share and rehabilitate.

The Ostomy visitor (OV) form a group along with the surgeon and stoma nurse for the well being of the patient who is undergoing ostomy.

## ■ THE OBJECTIVES OF OSTOMY VISITOR (FIG. 20.1 AND TABLE 20.1)

*   To learn the role and responsibilities of a visitor and basic visiting policies.
*   To recognise psychological and social issues of the ostomates.
*   To provide necessary inputs and information to the ostomates, as regards to acceptance of their own ostomy.

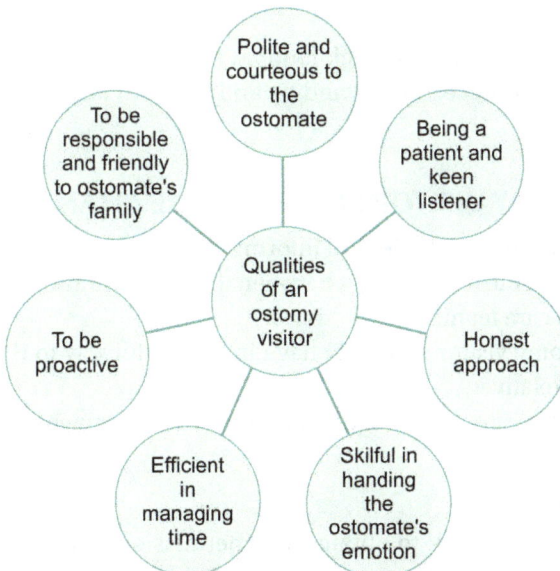

**Fig. 20.1:** Qualities of an ostomy visitor

**Table 20.1:** Types of visit

| | |
|---|---|
| Before surgery | • Before surgery, visits should be short<br>• To give basic answers to ostomate's questions.<br>• To refer any medical questions back to their doctor or nurse.<br>• To avoid talking about the operation.<br>• Offer to come back after the surgery.<br>• Not to talk about medical information. |
| After surgery in hospital | • To be sensitive to the fact that the ostomate may be medicated and therefore not as responsive.<br>• Respond quickly when asked to make a hospital visit.<br>• Make the visit short, limited to 15–30 minutes depending on the Ostomate's condition.<br>• Answer questions factually and to the limit of one's own experience. |
| At home | • A home visit is a more relaxed one.<br>• There may be more distractions in a home visit because of the family setting.<br>• The Ostomate may be feeling better and the visit is more relaxed.<br>• However, the home may be very busy with activities.<br>• The home visit may be an opportunity to include interested family members in the discussion |
| By telephone | • A telephone visit allows for a contact with the ostomate with no added stress on the ostomate or the visitor.<br>• Offer to meet the person in a follow up visit. |
| At support group meetings | Going to a support group might be helpful before surgery for some. For some new Ostomates, it may be the first opportunity to meet with other Ostomates. |

(*Courtesy*: http://win.fais.info/pdf/IOA_visitorguideline_English.pdf, page 9)

- To support ostomates and their families to adjust to living with stoma.
- To offer reassurance, understanding and practical information regarding the ostomy.

## ■ THE OSTOMY VISITOR SHOULD UNDERSTAND

- He or she is not to give medical information.
- Must respect the relationships between the ostomate and the members of the health care team.
- Every ostomy visitor should behave in respectful way to the ostomates and their relatives.
- The ostomy visitor is not required to show his or her own stoma.

## Permission

It is necessary for an OV to obtain prior permission from the ostomate or the health authority prior to a visit (*Courtesy*: http://win.fais.info/pdf/IOA_visitorguideline_English.pdf, page 8).

## Privacy

Ostomates' names are always kept confidential and should not be discussed with anyone outside the health care team.

## Medical Advice

An OV should not initiate discussion regarding the ostamate's diagnosis or give medical treatment advice. The OV should inform the doctor or stoma nurse about any requests by the ostomate for medical advice.

## Stoma Care

The OV should neither involve in the stoma care of the patient or should recommend any ostomy products.

The OV is not expected to talk too much about his or her own personal experience, but spend time listening to the ostomate.

The OV should not discuss religion, politics and other sensitive issues and is expected to respect the beliefs of the ostomate.

Before surgery, the visit should be short to give basic answers to Ostomates questions. For any medical queries, it is better to refer to ET nurse or doctor.

After the surgery, the OV when asked to make a visit should spend limited time depending on Ostomate's condition.

The OV can choose visiting the ostomate at hospital, home, depending on the convenience of the patient.

A telephone visit allows for contact with the ostomate with no added stress both for the ostomate and for the visitor.

## ■ BIBLIOGRAPHY

1. International Ostomy association-Visitor training guidelines-an IOA initiative. http://win.fais.info/pdf/IOA_visitorguideline_English.pdf

# Challenges Faced by Handicapped Ostomates

## ■ INTRODUCTION

In normal stoma patients the tasks of managing his or her stoma includes emptying and removing the pouching system, washing and drying the skin, measuring the stoma, putting a new pouching system and disposing of the used pouch system. These tasks are challenging to patients with the following physical and mental handicaps.

- Mental and sensory deficits like peripheral neuropathy, Parkinsonism, motor neuron disease, multiple sclerosis and stroke.
- Visual deficits like blindness and impaired vision.
- Joint diseases like Rheumatoid arthritis.

## ■ MENTAL ILLNESS

- Ostomates with mental illness may respond differently to ostomy
- They may fail to recognise regarding the emptying and changing of the appliance or they may frequently meddle with the stoma bag leading to peristomal skin damage and leakage.
- Some of the patients may have difficulty to learn about the self care.
- Yet other patients may consider this appliance as an alien to their body and would start attacking them causing harm to the body and peristomal skin.

## ■ VISUAL ILLNESS

In a visually handicapped ostomate their compromised eye sight can greatly hinder the ability of the ostomate to measure the stoma for an appliance, to see peristomal complications or to empty the pouch. This ultimately interferes in the self care management of stoma which can negatively influence body image.

## ■ MOTOR SENSORY ILLNESS

Ostomates with motor sensory deficits are handicapped with reduced ability to perform their duties with manual dexterity. So they are handicapped to manually resize and apply the pouch systems over the stoma.

Patients with advanced disease and terminal illness also have difficulty in managing their own stoma.

## ROLE OF WOCN AND ET NURSE

It is the duty of the wound ostomy continence nurse (WOCN) or enterostomal therapy nurse (ETN) to examine and identify the ostomate with regards to their physical and mental health including their illness and comorbid status.

Sometimes it becomes necessary to go into the details of the ostomates' history and rule out any other diseases or deformities or disorders before embarking on their care. The duties of WOCN and ETN in caring the ostomates with these physical and mental handicaps are complex and truly challenging. They have to perform tasks such as emptying and removing the pouching system, washing and drying the skin, measuring the stoma, putting a new pouching system and disposing of the used pouch system.

These patients may in addition have trouble shooting problems like leakage which has to be attended. These people are into medications for their own illness which has to be identified and carried out properly. More emphasis should be given in preventing the peristomal complications.

At last it is very important for the WOCN and ETN to teach and educate these ostomates and seek help whenever necessary from them.

## BIBLIOGRAPHY

1. Caring for the patient with fecal or urinary diversion
   http://www.o-wm.com/content/caring-patient-fecal-or-urinary-diversion-palliative-and-hospice-settings-literature-review

# Ostomy and Social Media

In today's world media plays a very important role in public life. It plays a very constructive role in bridging the society with various information and knowledge to people. It is one of the more powerful instruments of communication where one can learn loads of social problems and issues and can also share information of any kind to all people for better living.

However, because of freedom, the media is sometimes biased and may become liable so one has to choose the right one to get information. But one should not forget that the media has got a vital role in moulding a good society to develop our life style and move it on the right path.

As far as ostomy or stoma care is concerned in the media, there are several avenues available in the web.

## ■ FACEBOOK

Facebook is great because this is a forum wherein an ostomate can find (a) Support group pages, (b) Ostomate groups, (c) Product sellers information about group, (d) 24×7 stoma support group, (e) On call stoma nurses or WOCN, wherein one can get in touch with to attend to their problems and queries regarding their stoma and also seek their help in fixing the stoma appliance and clarifying their doubts regarding the same.

An Ostomate can make friends through online with another ostomy person who can give them confidence, boost up their moral, build positive energy in mind and get to know the help and information from them.

## ■ TWITTER

It is one of the favorite social media platforms wherein, an ostomate can find people out there who are experiencing the same thing what they face. One can seek their advice by creating a blog about their issue. For example "My stoma site is really sore", "My bag keeps leaking". With a quick tweet sent to the twitter sphere, immediately there are lots of advices and informations pouring into the media.

Twitter also provides quick updates about medical and appliance advances as well as campaigns regarding ostomy world. Hence twitter inspires an ostomate to keep in touch with the ostomy community.

## ▣ YOUTUBE

This is an excellent visual platform for an ostomate to learn anything and everything about ostomy care. This site conveys all the information through videos, that an ostomate needs regarding

- Lifestyle tips
- Stoma care
- Continence care
- How to use the products in terms of ostomy care
- Tips from health care professionals like the physicians, surgeons who are connected to the ostomy service
- Informations and contact details about ET nurse.

There is exhausting information about the stoma products available in Youtube produced by the different supplier groups like Hollister, Convatec, Coloplast and Prowess.

This site also provides information regarding the disease profile that an ostomate suffers.

## ▣ WEBSITES OFFERING STOMA CARE

- There are number of websites available worldwide to offer information regarding solutions for stoma care.
- About different products available from different sources of manufacturer
- Tips to live with a stoma
- Volunteer based health organisations offering mutual aid and moral support to the ostomates
- Education information for ostomy and stoma care

## ▣ BIBLIOGRAPHY

1. Never underestimate the power of social media-SecuriCare
   http://www.securicaremedical.co.uk/Menu/Securicare-Blog/ArtMID/15413/ArticleID/56/Social-media-and-stoma.aspx

# Ostomy Supplies and Agencies in Ostomy Care

There are several manufacturers mostly from around the world and a few products from India which are marketed for stoma care. The following are the companies that supply to the Indian market:

| Manufacturer/name | Service | Website |
|---|---|---|
| B.Braun India | Products-stoma care for education of ostomates and easy use of their products | www.bbraun.co.in |
| Hollister | This is an ostomy care company which manufactures all categories of stoma care products | www.hollister.com |
| Coloplast | This company has a dedicated service for the end users with the stoma. They have a wide range of products for ostomy care. | www. coloplast.com |
| Convatec India Pvt. Ltd. | It is an international provider of medical products and technologies offering products and services for ostomy care | www.convatec.co.in |
| Prowess stoma care | This is a leading Indian manufacturer with state-of-the art ostomy products. | www.prowesscare.com |
| Ostomy service | This Chennai based Indian company specialises in personalised services with counseling. They also provide hospital and house visits providing support to the patients and to their relatives about the stoma care and the application of the pouches. They also supply the stoma care products. | www.stomacare.co.in |

## ■ BIBLIOGRAPHY

1. http://www.colostomyassociation.org.uk/
2. https://www.ncbi.nlm.nih.gov/pmc/articles/PMC1963634/
3. https://www.coloplast.in/stoma/
4. http://www.dchft.nhs.uk/patients/departments-PZ/Pages/Stoma-Care.aspx
5. www.bbraun.co.in
6. www.hollister.com
7. www. coloplast.com
8. www.convatec.co.in

CHAPTER

**24**

# Ostomy Associations in India and Abroad

## ■ INTRODUCTION

There are number of Ostomy associations in India and across the Globe which provides all the information necessary for ostomy care and service.

## ■ OSTOMY ASSOCIATION OF INDIA (OAI)

This is located in Mumbai and also at AIIMS, New Delhi, India. Its objectives are:

- To provide useful and helpful information to ostomates through literature, periodical meeting between the old ostomates and new ostomates to exchange the experience among themselves.
- To help to lead a normal physical, psychological and social life.
- To encourage formation of local clubs of ostomates in different parts of India.
- To educate nurse, doctors and the lay public in the requirements of the ostomates.
- To improve the management techniques to be taught to the ostomates and procure and make available suitable equipments for them.

## ■ OSTOMATES INDIA

This is situated in Bangalore, India, which deals with all the informations to ostomates and also provides necessary information about the ostomy products and their availability.

## ■ OSTOMY SERVICE

This is an information site about the development of ostomy service and the people who are involved in the service of ostomy care. Their website also provides detailed information about the ostomy appliances, availability of the services of WOCN and ETN and demo videos about different appliances.

## ■ UNITED OSTOMY ASSOCIATION OF AMERICA (UOAA)

- It is the place for ostomy resources, advocacy and support
- It is a member of International Ostomy Association

### ■ INTERNATIONAL OSTOMY ASSOCIATION (IOA)

The International Ostomy Association (IOA) is a non-profit federation of over 60 ostomy associations committed to improving the quality of life of individuals with ostomies and other related surgeries.

The International Ostomy Association is committed to encouraging the highest possible standards of surgery, medical attention, and patient after-care and assisting member organizations in helping affected individuals achieve the quality of life they seek after such surgical procedures. The aims of the association include providing information and management guidelines to member associations, helping to form new ostomy associations, and representing the interests of all individuals who receive ostomies and related surgeries.

### ■ COLOSTOMY ASSOCIATION

The Colostomy Association is a UK charity that provides support, reassurance and practical advice to anyone who has or is about to have stoma surgery.

They provide a wide range of informative booklets, quarterly magazine and Facebook support group reaching to anyone affected by stoma surgery.

### ■ AUSTRALIAN COUNCIL OF STOMA ASSOCIATIONS INC

The Australian Council of Stoma Associations Inc represents, at a national level, the interests of 22 regional Stoma Associations located throughout Australia.

They encourage visitors to explore all areas of their site to gain a better understanding of the world of "ostomy".

### ■ WOUND, OSTOMY AND CONTINENCE NURSES SOCIETY (WOCN)

It is a professional, international nursing society of more than 5,000 health care professionals who are experts in the care of patients with wound, ostomy and incontinence. WOCN members serve as content experts, educators, and advisers in collaborative health initiatives to assure access to a WOC specialty practice nurse.

### ■ GOLD COAST OSTOMY ASSOCIATION (GCOA)

The Gold Coast Ostomy Association is an organisation which provides support, information and advocacy to Ostomates and their care givers. It also facilitates member Ostomate access to stoma appliances and pharmaceutical benefit products pursuant to the provisions of the national Stoma Appliance

Scheme. The Association is also a proud member of the Australian Council of Stoma Associations ( ACSA ).

## ■ THE DANISH OSTOMY ASSOCIATION COPA

The Ostomy Association COPA is the world's oldest patient association for persons with ostomy.

Its objectives are:
- To make the situation better for ostomy/pouch operated and people with other diseases in the intestines.
- To serve as a mouthpiece for all ostomy patients when facing the public health system.
- To provide free help and advice to people before, during and/or after their hospitalization on topics like "how to live a normal life with an ostomy"..
- To help other countries build ostomy associations, and give practical help, by sending spare ostomy products to help those who are in need.
- COPA has its own website (www.copa.dk)

## ■ BIBLIOGRAPHY

1. http://www.ostomy.org/Home.html
2. http://www.ostomyinternational.org/
3. https://rarediseases.org/organizations/international-ostomy-association/
4. https://www.goldcoastostomy.com.au/news/
5. International Ostomy Association-NORD

# Amazing Ostomates

| | |
|---|---|
| | **Napoleon Bonaparte**<br>Military conqueror and a world leader. |
| | **Dwight Eisenhower**<br>Former president of the United States. |
| | **Marvin Bush**<br>Former US President George W Bush's son |
| | **Richard Bernard Skelton or "Red Skelton'**<br>One of the great American Entertainers and National television and Radio comedian |
| | **Jerry Kramer**<br>Former American football player. |

Before I bring to your notice, the amazing Ostomates whom I have come across at Chennai, TN, India, I wish to tell you about the "World Ostomy Day" which is meant to improve the rehabilitation of the ostomates world wide by bringing to the attention of the general public and the global community the needs and aspirations of the ostomates.

There are many stories but there is only one voice, it is the voice of the ostomates that has to be listened to, to help them.

The world ostomy day is celebrated across the world through educational programs, seminars, supporting meetings and demonstrations in the first week of October every year.

I have come across some amazing ostomates who have stoma, yet leading a very happy and prosperous life

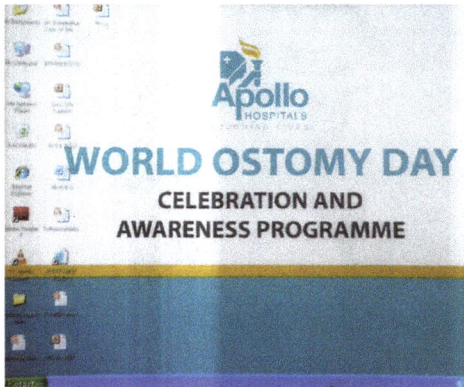

World Ostomy Day celebrations at Apollo Hospitals, Chennai

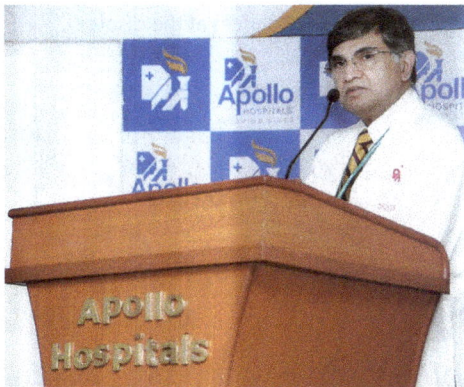

Dr KS Prasanna Kumar Reddy addressing at the World Ostomy Day

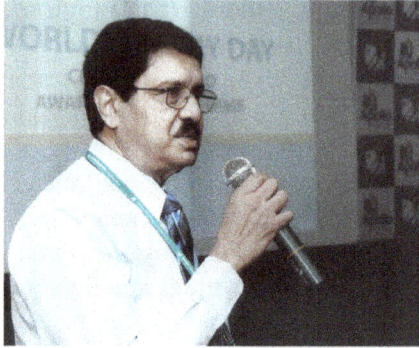

Author addressing on World Ostomy Day

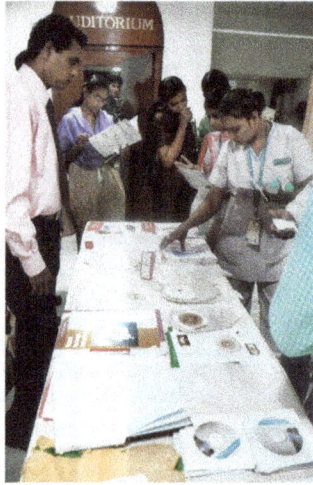

Ostomy appliances at the display

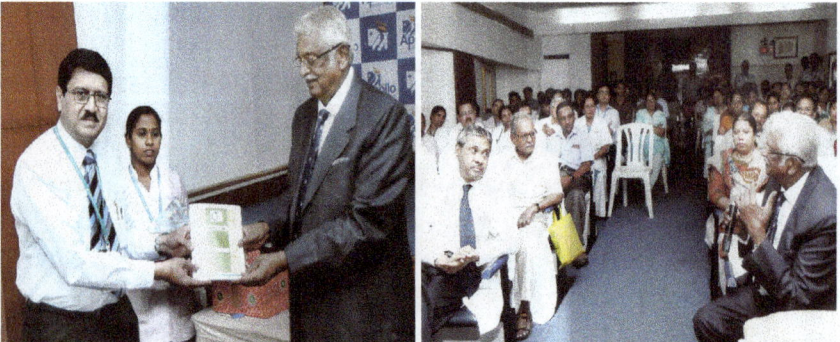

Late Professor N Rangabashyam receiving the 1st copy of a booklet on Stoma care written by the author, followed by addressing the gathering on the issues related to Stoma care

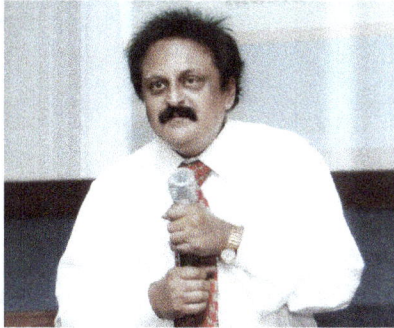

Underwent permanent ileostomy following ulcerative colitis. Successful personality development trainer who has achieved remarkably even after having an Ostomy

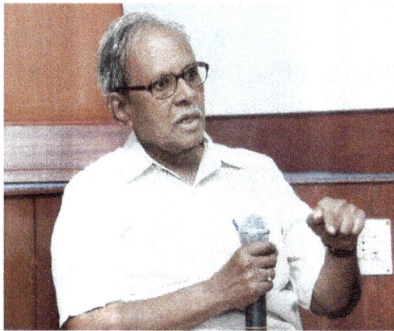

A 78-year-old, has ileal urinary conduit following removal of his urinary bladder due to cancer. Highly spirited and volunteers himself as an Ostomy visitor and a social care provider.

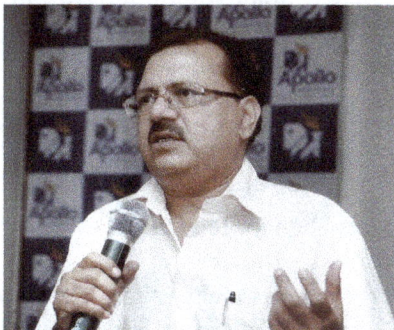

An industrialist by profession. Underwent permanent ileostomy for ulcerative colitis. His Ostomy has never altered his way of life.

## ◼ BIBLIOGRAPHY

1. http://www.shieldhealthcare.com/community/ostomylife/2016/03/29/famous-people-with-ostomies/

# Frequently Asked Questions

## ■ INTRODUCTION

Following stoma forming surgery, patients will have many questions about the stoma and how it might affect their lifestyle, work and social activities. Some of the questions commonly asked by patients are discussed in this chapter. The advice outlined in the answers is general in nature and if you have any doubts or concerns about an individual patient's queries it is essential that you involve the stoma care nurse (SCN). Equally, if patients have specific concerns regarding their stoma management or surgery you should advise the patient to discuss these with their SCN or the consultant who performed their surgery as they will be able to advise the patient more specifically, bearing in mind the underlying condition and the surgical procedure performed.

## ■ COMMONLY ASKED QUESTIONS

Patients have many information needs and will be given a large amount of information at all stages of their treatment. This information will be both written and verbal but will require reinforcement and clarification. The majority of appliance manufacturers and national ostomy support groups produce booklets summarizing the basics of stoma surgery and stoma management. Such booklets are available in the stoma care clinic, Department of Surgical Gastroenterology, Apollo Hospitals, Greams road, Chennai.

### Will I have to alter my diet or avoid certain foods?

Following stoma surgery patients often think they will have to totally change their diet and severely restrict their food intake. This is not the case but patients need to be aware of minor alterations that they may need to make to their food and fluid input following surgery. When discussing food with patients, try to avoid using the term 'diet' as this can be interpreted negatively by many patients as meaning rigid restrictions to their diet or that they have to be on a 'special diet' now that they have a stoma. The main concern for ostomists is that certain foods can cause a change in stool consistency or an increase in wind and odor. It is essential that ostomists experiment with their food intake and do not exclude an item from their diet after having tried it once only. Initially after surgery many foods may cause increased wind but after a few months many ostomists find they can eat what they perceived initially to be problematic foods with no problems. Therefore, the key to a healthy diet for the ostomist is experimentation with food. Rigid instructions are impossible to give as everybody reacts differently to and likes different foods. There are NO foods which MUST be avoided or excluded from the ostomist's diet.

## General dietary tips for the ostomist

- Chew food thoroughly.
- Try to eat three meals a day at regular times.
- Drink a minimum of eight cups of fluid per day.
- Ensure fruit and vegetables are included in the diet.
- When trying new foods for the first time after surgery try a small portion first and then gradually increase to a normal size serving.
- If on first eating a food causes wind, do not exclude it from your diet, wait a few weeks and then try again.

*Foods which can cause excess wind formation in the Ostomist with a fecal stoma include:*

| *Beer* | *Brussel sprouts* | *Cabbage* |
|---|---|---|
| Cauliflower | Cucumber | Eggs |
| Beans | Onions | Spicy foods |

The following that can help to reduce wind production are as follows:
- Do not talk while eating.
- Avoid drinking through a straw.
- Avoid fizzy drinks (pour drinks into a glass to get rid of some of the bubbles and let it stand for five minutes or so before drinking).
- Eat regularly and do not miss meals.
- Eat slowly.
- Natural yoghurt.
- Peppermint tea.
  For a colostomist, there are really no dietary restrictions but the ileostomist should be aware of a number of issues:
- An ileostomist will lose more water and salt through their ileostomy output than prior to their surgery (as they no longer reabsorb water from the colon) and therefore they will need to drink around eight to ten cups of fluid per day to make up for this loss, equally they will need to add extra salt to their food on the plate and use salt in cooking.

- Certain foods which are very high in fiber and poorly digested can temporarily 'block' the stoma. Therefore, all high fiber foods such as nuts, celery, and sweet corn should be chewed well.

For the urostomist, there is no special dietary advice but there are some guidelines regarding their fluid and food intake:

- Fish and asparagus can give the urine an unusual odor.
- A glass of cranberry juice a day can reduce the amount of mucus produced by the stoma.
- Foods high in vitamin C (such as oranges) can help to keep the urine more acid which can help prevent urinary tract infections.
- If the urine appears dark it is a sign that the urine is becoming concentrated and the urostomist needs to drink more fluid to ensure the urine remains dilute.

## Can I drink alcohol now that i have a stoma?

Alcohol can be included as part of a healthy diet for all ostomists. Gassy drinks such as beer can cause wind. It is advisable to adhere to the recommended alcohol intake of 2 to 3 units per day for women and 3 to 4 units per day for men. Regular consumption above this recommended level becomes detrimental to health. One unit of alcohol is equal to 1 pub measure of spirit or half a pint of beer/lager.

It is not advisable to save up units to have 'a big night out'. If the ostomist does overindulge they may have problems with emptying or changing the appliance, which could cause leakage or spillage problems.

## Can I play sports?

Generally patients should be advised to avoid strenuous exercise and lifting for 6 weeks after their operation to allow the wound to fully heal, but during this time walking is a good and safe form of exercise. There is a risk of incisional hernia formation following any abdominal surgery and therefore it is important that patients do not commence strenuous exercise or lifting prior to this to ensure that the abdominal muscles have fully healed. Once the patient has been reviewed by their surgeon in the outpatient department, usually 6 to 8 weeks after their operation, they will be given the all clear to start exercising fully again. Participation in contact sports is possible with a stoma but it is important to avoid any direct trauma to the stoma. A plastic stomal cap is available, which protects the stoma from trauma. This is placed over the stoma, on top of the appliance and is held in place by an elasticated belt. The SCN can arrange a stomal cap for patients and will advise on its use. Swimming is a good exercise, it is advisable for patients to eat lightly prior to swimming and ensure the pouch is emptied just before swimming. There are a variety of small pouches which are ideal for sporting activities, and the SCN can supply samples of these for patients to try. There is also a range of swimwear with internal pockets to both support and disguise the appliance. A number of companies manufacture these, and again the SCN can provide the appropriate details. For those who engage in vigorous exercise there are additional belts which may be worn to support the stoma and the appliance. If the patient has any doubts at all they should discuss their concerns with the SCN prior to commencing any new sporting activities.

## Can I wear my normal clothes?

It is advisable for patients to wear snug fitting underclothes. If the appliance is placed inside the pants it supports the pouch and prevents movement of the appliance when the patient moves. Modification to clothing should be minimal if at all. It is important that belts or very firm waistbands do not cross directly over the stoma as this may cause trauma to the stoma. If the waistband lies directly over the stoma men may be advised to wear braces and not a belt. Some patients will slightly alter their style of dress, e.g. by wearing skirts or trousers with front pleats to disguise the stoma. It is fine for women to wear tights and if they wish to wear a tight fitting panty girdle these can be made specifically for them with an aperture for the appliance so that the fecal/urinary output can flow into the appliance freely. These girdles can be arranged through the SCN. The patient will quite naturally need time to rebuild confidence in their body image and at first may restrict themselves to baggy clothing. Initially this may be more comfortable because of the abdominal wound but patients should be encouraged to try their normal clothing. Should it be necessary, several manufacturers have designed items of clothing specifically for the ostomist, e.g. high-waisted trousers. The SCN will be able to give the patient specific information about these items. Once wearing their normal clothing, patients quickly realize that the appliance is not noticeable and this will of course help to boost their confidence and self-esteem.

## Can I go back to work?

The majority of patients can return to their work environment. After stoma forming surgery, it is reasonable to assume that as long as the patient is not undergoing any further treatment (such as chemotherapy) they should be able to return to work in approximately 12—16 weeks. Patients should be advised to keep an 'emergency' supply of all items required for a bag change at work.

Often patients are worried about changing or emptying their appliance in a public toilet. Many patients are worried about leaving 'tell-tale' odors in the toilet and the SCN can provide the patient with a deodoriser to ensure this concern is minimized. If the patient's occupation involves rigorous activity or heavy lifting the patient should consult their doctor prior to returning to work.

## Can I take my pouch off in the bath or shower?

It is safe for patients to remove their appliance before bathing and showering. Often patients are concerned that bathwater will enter the stoma but this is not the case. It is a matter of personal choice for patients but if they choose to keep the appliance on during bathing the appliance will need to be patted dry with a towel afterwards. Appliances are waterproof and the security of the adhesive is not reduced if it gets wet.

## Where do I get my supplies?

While in hospital all the patient's stoma supplies will be provided by the SCN. The SCN will arrange for the patient to obtain the supplies from the supplier or from the ostomy care center. At home patients have a choice of how they order their supplies once they have a prescription. They can take the prescription to a chemist; supplies will not be in stock but will be obtained by the chemist within a couple of days. Alternatively, they may use a home delivery service by contacting the suppliers or the chemist or carry bulky supplies home, equally many home delivery companies will arrange repeat prescriptions directly with the patient's GP. If the patient feels they would like to use a home delivery service the SCN can arrange the supply from the stoma clinics in Apollo hospital or from the stoma supply dealers.

## How do I dispose of my used stoma appliance?

The recommended method of disposal is to empty the contents of the appliance down the toilet, seal the used appliance in a plastic bag and place it in the household bin.

## Can I go away on holiday?

Patients often worry about managing their stoma away from their home environment and will need encouragement and reassurance. Often just talking through their concerns will be enough to reassure them. There is no reason why a person with a stoma may not travel abroad or take a holiday. There are travel certificates available in many languages explaining that the patient has a medical condition and is carrying medical supplies in their hand luggage. This is particularly useful at Customs and avoids embarrassing bag searches. This certificate is available from the SCN. Patients should be advised to take double the amount of equipment that they would normally use for that period of time (to allow for any emergencies or increased appliance changes caused by travelers' diarrhea) and to ensure it is carried in their hand luggage. This avoids any worries about luggage not arriving with the patient at their destination. The only potential problem with flying is that everybody tends to produce more wind due to the changes in cabin pressure.

Avoiding fizzy drinks while on the journey that can help to minimize the wind production and the use of an appliance with a flatus filter can avoid the appliance filling with wind. It might be advisable to book an aisle seat to allow easy access to the toilets during the flight. As with any traveler there is a risk of 'travelers' diarrhea' caused by the change in climate, food and water in a foreign country. Patients should be advised to drink bottled water and to increase their water and salt consumption in hot weather. Avoid ice cubes and salads, which may have been washed in tapwater. Highly spiced foods should be treated with some caution especially if the patient is not used to eating them at home. If diarrhea is a problem while on holiday the advice to an ostomist would be very similar to the general advice anyone would receive:

- Drink plenty of water to replace what's being lost.
- Replace the salt and potassium lost by adding salt to food and drink fruit juices and savoury drinks. Over-the-counter oral rehydration products can be used.
- Use an antidiarrheal drug which can now be bought over-the-counter at the chemist shops.

With regard to travel insurance it is essential that patients check with their insurer to ensure that pre-existing medical conditions are not excluded from the insurance. The relevant ostomy support group will be able to advise on suitable travel insurance companies.

## When can I drive again?

Patients can usually resume driving 6 to 8 weeks after surgery. Normally the surgeon will say that once a patient feels they are able to do an emergency stop it is safe for them to drive. It usually takes about 6 weeks for the patient to feel comfortable to do this and you can suggest that once a patient can stamp their foot with no abdominal pain they can drive. Patients may be concerned about the seat belt rubbing on the stoma. Products are available that hold the seat belt away from the abdomen (therefore stopping any friction/rubbing on the stoma). These can be bought from car accessory shops.

## Are there any support groups available for people with a stoma?

In India we have the OstomatesIndia. There are a number of both national and local support groups and charities. The SCN will ensure that the patient is fully aware of the groups which are appropriate to them. Membership of these organizations that can provide many benefits for patients, not least of these are social interaction and peer support. These organizations also produce very informative newsletters and information sheets, members are sent these periodically and they help to keep patients up-to-date especially regarding the availability and development of new stoma products. Ostomy Association of India is providing equipment to urostomy, colostomy ileostomy management and counseling the new patient. Ostomy Association of India procures ostomy equipments manufactured in India or Imported, and they are supplied to the Ostomates on No-profit No- Loss Basis. For outstation members equipments are sent by parcel. Meet the ostomates and learn about their association. Mr T Singaravel can be contacted at 22031082. This is part of the HELP Talk Series At HELP, Health Education Library For People, The Worlds Largest Free Patient Education Library. www.healthlibrarv.com. Another is ostomatesindiawhich is present in Bangalore, at 1308, 11th B Cross, Vyalikaval, Bangalore - 560003. E-mail: ostomates_india@yahoo.co.in. Ostomates India's Phone Numbers, Phone: - 23386229 with more than 10,000 members and 12 branches in india. They conduct free checkups from 11 am to 4 pm on first saturdays of the month.

## Who should I tell about my stoma?

One of the main concerns for the ostomist is the issue of 'Who to tell' and 'How to tell' about their stoma. Initially patients may only wish their partner/close family members to know. As a person becomes more confident in the management of their stoma and begins to resume their usual social and work activities they may wish to tell others about their stoma. There is no right or wrong way to do this and often patients find it useful to role-play the discussion they wish to have. This is something that the SCN will be able to facilitate and support. The key to remember is that if something is presented positively and without embarrassment that is how it will be perceived by the person receiving the news. The young person without an established sexual relationship will need advice on how and when to tell their new 'partner' about the stoma. If social interaction is severely curtailed because of 'fear' of the stoma referral to other sources of advice such as psychosexual counselors may be beneficial.

## Can I still have sexual intercourse?

Naturally many ostomists are anxious about resuming sexual activity. Much of this anxiety stems from concerns about their change in body image and attractiveness to their partner. Reassurance should be given that sexual activity will not hurt the stoma. Practical suggestions can be given to the patient to reduce anxiety such as:

- Empty the appliance prior to sexual activity.
- Use of a small appliance, stomal cap or appliance cover can lessen the presence of the appliance.
- The appliance may be rolled up to make it smaller and taped down so that it does not move. Men may have concerns about or problems with impotence due to damage to the nerves during pelvic surgery. This can be discussed with the surgeon; many options are now available to treat this problem. Women may experience discomfort on deep penenetration and the SCN will be able to discuss with them changes in sexual positions or the use of extra vaginal lubricants. Initially concerns about sexual activity center around issues regarding the change in the body image following surgery. Following major abdominal surgery it is likely that many patients will experience a decrease in libido. As their general health improves, for many so does their libido and it is at this stage that the SCN will be able to answer questions they might have and support the patient and their partner to be open in discussing their concerns and feelings. Patients often find it easier to discuss these intimate concerns with the SCN with whom they have developed a trusting relationship and therefore any concerns or issues raised by the patient are often best referred to the SCN.

## Can I become pregnant now I have had a stoma?

Women with a stoma can become pregnant and have a normal pregnancy. Patients requiring contraception or wishing to discuss conception would be best advised to see their consultant or general practitioner (GP). Patients with an ileostomy may not be able to use the oral contraceptive pill as it may be excreted without being fully absorbed. Any surgery to the pelvic floor can alter the anatomy, which may make the use of the intrauterine device (IUD) or cap which is difficult. Some women who have had severe pelvic sepsis (Crohn's disease) may experience fertility problems but for the majority of women with a stoma fertility is unaffected. Some women may be advised by their obstetrician to have a cesarian section.

## What can I do to prevent odour?

Without doubt this is the most common worry of patients with a stoma. Modern appliances are made of layers of bonded plastic and are odor proof. If the flange becomes displaced or the seal is detached, odor will escape from the bag. During an appliance change or emptying of the appliance there will be odor but the patients need to be reassured that this is taking place in the toilet/bathroom where people usually open their bowels and there is odor. Domestic air fresheners mask odor and are commonly used in toilets/ bathrooms. There are also deodoriser sprays available, which leave no odour. Patients have reported that striking a match in the toilet dispels odor. The matchstick can then be flushed down the toilet leaving no evidence. Alongside the deodoriser sprays the SCN can suggest and are available on prescription are a number of drops/pellets which can be placed in the appliance prior to use and help deodorise once emptied. Flatus filters allow air to come out of the appliance so that it does not distend and become visible. These are made of charcoal to deodorise the flatus as it leaves the appliance so no tell-tale odor is noticeable.

## Now that I have a stoma will anything come out of my back passage?

The answer to this question will depend entirely on the type of surgery the patient has had. If they have had an abdominoperineal excision of rectum and formation of colostomy or a panproctocolectomy their rectum and anus has been surgically removed and therefore there is no remaining orifice. If patients still have part of their rectum or anus they will continue to pass mucus (the bowel's natural lubricant). They can often have the sensation of wanting to have their bowels open and should be advised to sit on the toilet and push gently to expel any mucus. If they do this once or twice a day it will prevent a buildup of mucus and therefore prevent the sensation of wanting to have their bowels open. If the patient has a loop (or double-barrel stoma) it is possible for some fecal matter to by-pass the appliance and pass into the defuctioned loop of bowel. This occurs rarely but may result in the patient passing small amounts of stool per rectum.

## Will any medicines I take affect the way my stoma works?

Many drugs can affect stomal function and some medications will not be completely absorbed. Patients should be advised to discuss this issue with their stoma care nurse (SCN) or General practioner (GP) prior to commencing any new medications.

Drug possible effect on stoma. Antibiotics may cause diarrhea as they interfere with normal gut flora and cause the effluent to be green in color. Anti-depressants may cause constipation in colostomy patients. Laxatives anti-psychotics and/or stool softeners may be used in conjunction with these drugs. Analgesics may cause constipation and often laxatives and/or stool containing softeners may be used in conjunction in the colostomist codeine/ opiates. Any enteric- Probably ineffective particularly in the ileostomist as not coated or fully absorbed sustained-release drug. Iron will darken the color of the stool to black. Antacids may make colostomy and ileostomy output gray in color. Amitriptyline can cause urine to have a blue-green color. Metronidazole can turn urine a reddish-brown color Senna can turn urine yellow/brown. Warfarin can turn urine orange.

## ■ BIBLIOGRAPHY

1. FAQs-Stoma-Clinimed
   http://www.clinimed.co.uk/Stoma-Care/FAQs.aspx
2. Frequently asked questions following stoma surgery
   http://www.eakincohesiveseals.com/frequently-asked-questions-following-stoma-surgery
3. Ostomy FAQ- The stolen colon Living beautifully with an Ostomy
   http://stolencolon.com/ostomy-faq/
4. Ostomy FAQ-United Ostomy Association of America Inc.
   http://www.ostomy.org/Ostomy_FAQ.html
5. Ostomy FAQs-Questions and answers about having an Ostomy
   https://www.veganostomy.ca/ostomy-faqs/
6. Your "How to" Ostomy tips
   http://www.premiersystems.net/ostomates.pdf

# Glossary of Terms

| | |
|---|---|
| **Adhesions** | Scar tissue from an abdominal surgery can generate adhesions which are fibrous bands that may attach to the bowel. These can sometimes cause blockages in the intestine, though this is a rare occurrence. |
| **Appliance** | The formal term for an ostomy pouch or ostomy bag. |
| **Anti-reflux valve** | A valve incorporated in urostomy appliances. This valve stops the urine from going back into the kidneys once it has drained into the pouch. |
| **Ascending colostomy** | Ascending colostomy<br><br>A relatively rare opening in the ascending portion of the colon. It is located on the right side of the abdomen. |
| **Belts** | <br>Stoma belt<br>One of the accessories of stoma products. |
| **Colectomy** | The surgical removal of the colon (also known as the large intestine), often due to cancer, or noncancerous conditions such as severe inflammatory bowel disease or ruptured diverticulitis. |
| **Colostomy** | The surgically constructed opening where a portion of the colon is brought through the abdominal wall to its skin surface. Colostomies can be further defined in the terms of construction ,location and permanence. |

| | |
|---|---|
| **Continent ileostomy (Kock Pouch)** | 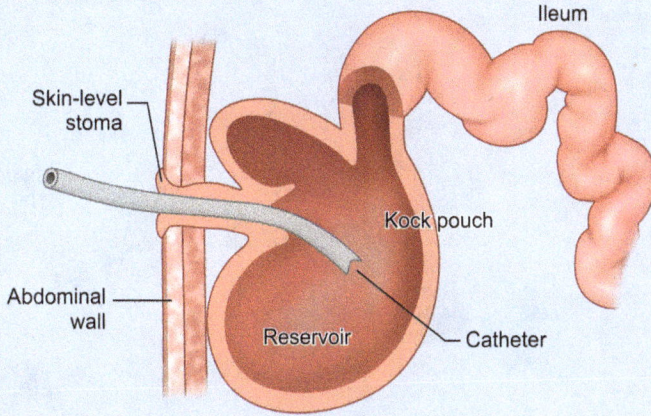 In this surgical variation of the ileostomy, a reservoir pouch is created inside the abdomen with a portion of the terminal ileum. A valve is constructed in the pouch and a stoma is brought through the abdominal wall. A catheter or tube is inserted into the pouch several times a day to drain feces from the reservoir. |
| **Continent urostomy** | 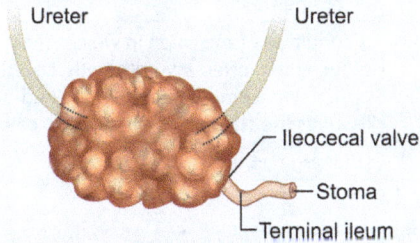 Indiana pouch: Pouch is made from larger interstine (ascending colon). Natural ileocecal valve is used for valve outlet made from terminal ileum<br><br>There are two main continent procedure alternatives to the ileal or cecal conduit (others exist). In both the Indiana and Kock pouch versions, a reservoir or pouch is created inside the abdomen using a portion of either the small or large bowel. A valve is constructed in the pouch and a stoma is brought through the abdominal wall. A catheter or tube is inserted several times daily to drain urine from the reservoir. |
| **Convexity** | Surface that is curved or rounded outward; provides tension on the skin, flattening peristomal skin contours causing a stoma to protrude better can be integrated (part of the barrier) or added (barrier rings). |

| | |
|---|---|
| **Crohn's disease** | <br>Intramural layer of fat and thickened walls<br><br>Inflammation and ulceration usually of the terminal portion of the ileum and/or small bowel. |
| **Diversion** | Surgical creation of an alternative route for effluent of the gastrointestinal (GI) tract, or of the urinary tract that can be described as 'continent or Incontinent'. |
| **Diverticulitis** | A condition of the colon in which small sacs or pouches form in the wall of the colon, often asymptomatic. Diverticulitis occurs when these small pouches become inflamed. Ruptured or perforated diverticulitis often requires the creation of a temporary colostomy. |
| **Effluent** | Discharge urine or stool. |
| **End ostomy construction** | <br>End colostomy<br><br>An ostomy in which the proximal cut end of the colon is formed into a stoma and the distal colon is either resected or closed. |

| | |
|---|---|
| **Enterostomal Therapy Nurse (ETN)** | Registered nurse who has advanced knowledge and clinical skill preparation from a recognized educational certificate program in the management of ostomies, wound and incontinence. |
| **Faceplate** | The part of the pouching system that adheres to the skin around the stoma. The faceplate can be separate from a pouch (two-piece system), or a pouch and faceplate can be one unit (one-piece system). |
| **Familial Adenomatous Polyposis (FAP)** | A hereditary disorder that is characterized by the development of multiple polyps (growths) in the colon. |
| **Flange** | A plastic ring on the faceplate (wafer) that allows a pouch to snap onto the faceplate. |
| **Flush stoma** | A stoma that is level with the skin. |
| **Folliculitis** | Folliculitis<br>An inflammation of the hair follicles occurring on one's skin around the stoma due to the physical trauma or as a result of frequent shaving of the skin around the stoma resulting in a rash or eruptions of the skin. |

| Hartman's procedure | 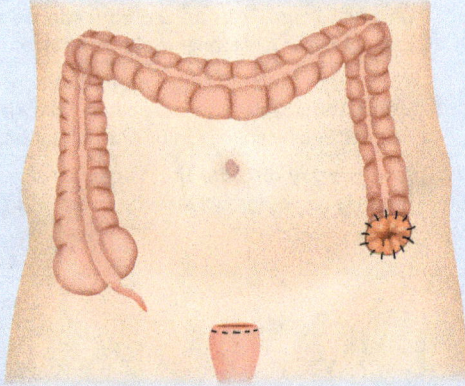 |
| --- | --- |
| | The surgical removal of a diseased portion of the distal colon or proximal rectum with formation of an end colostomy accompanied by over sewing of the distal colonic or rectal remnant. |
| Hernia parastomal | 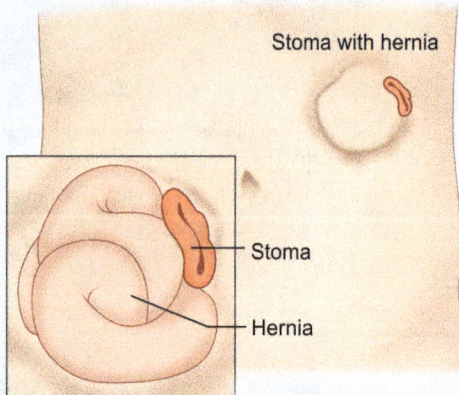<br>Stoma with hernia<br><br>Stoma<br><br>Hernia |
| | It occurs as a defect in the fascia that allows loops of intestine to protrude into the area of weakness. During stoma creation an opening is made into the fascia to allow the intestine to be advanced. In some patients this defect can enlarge, allowing the intestine to bulge into the area. May be supported with a wide belt or may require surgical correction. |

| Ileal conduit (Urostomy) | 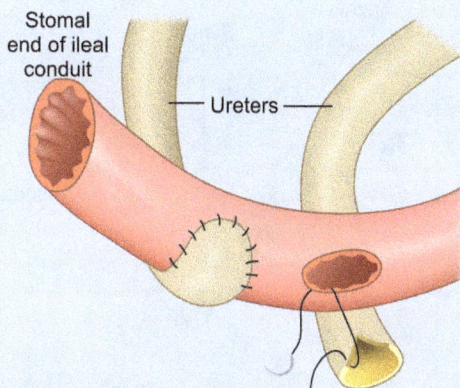 |
| --- | --- |
| | It is the most common urostomy. It is a method of diverting the urinary flow by transplanting the ureters into a prepared and isolated segment of the Ileum which is sutured and closed on one end. |
| Ileostomy | 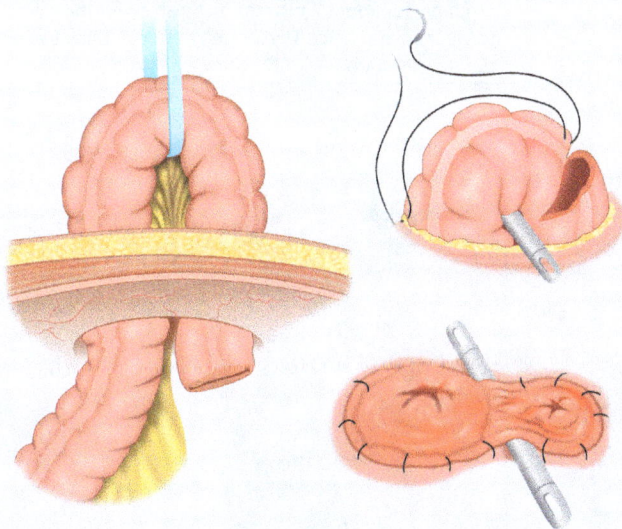 |
| | A surgical passage through the abdominal wall through which a segment of Ileum is exteriorized. An end stoma or loop stoma may be created. |
| Inflammatory bowel disease | The term for a number of chronic relapsing diseases of the gastrointestinal tract of unknown etiology. |

| Irrigation |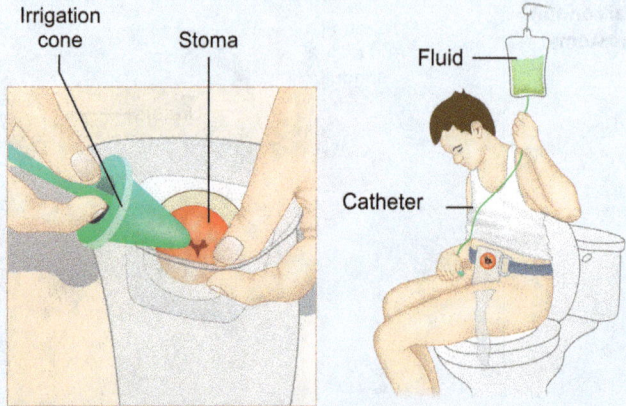

A procedure that people with colostomies undertake to regulate their bowel movements. This process is much like taking an enema. It's typically performed every day or every other day. After irrigating regularly for about 2 months, the person with a colostomy may not need to wear an appliance any longer, as the colon is 'trained' to only eliminate during irrigation. |
|---|---|
| Karaya |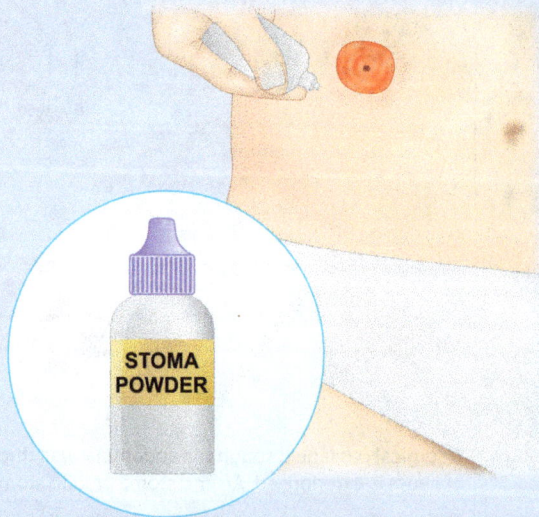

A vegetable based natural product recognized as safe and non-toxic. It can absorb as much as 100 times its weight in water forming a gel or paste that can be used to comfortably and safely smooth out rough or uneven skin. As an ostomy supply it is available in powder, paste and gel form. |
| Loop ostomy creation | Usually created in the transverse colon. It can be constructed in the small and large bowel. This is one stoma with two openings; one discharges stool and the other mucous. |

| | |
|---|---|
| **Obstruction** | A partial or complete blockage of small or large intestine. |
| **Ostomy** | A surgical procedure creating an opening between the urinary or GI tract and the skin. |
| **Ostomy-Temporary** | Usually the surgical plan is to reconnect the intestine and to close the ostomy. |
| **Ostomy-Permanent** | Ostomy that will never be closed. |
| **Peristomal candidiasis** | The overgrowth of a Candida organism of sufficient magnitude to cause inflammation, infection or disease on the skin of peristomal plane. |
| **Peristomal (Allergic) contact Dermatitis** | Any inflammation of the skin believed to be due to an allergic reaction to one or more components of a product (pouching systems and/or accessories). |
| **Peristomal (irritant) contact Dermatitis** | Skin damage resulting from contact with fecal or urinary leakage. |
| **Peristomal skin/plane** | 3 to 4 inches of skin surface surrounding an abdominal stoma. |
| **Permanent Colostomy** | Usually involves the loss of part of the colon, most commonly the rectum. The end of the remaining portion of the colon is brought out to the abdominal wall to form the stoma. |
| **Pouch (Appliance, Bag)** | A waterproof receptacle that collects effluent (i.e. urine or stool). |
| **Pouching systems (Ostomy pouching systems)** | Composed of a skin barrier and a collection device to collect drainage (effluent). |
| **Prolapse** | <br><br>Occurs when the stoma no longer adheres correctly to where it comes out of the abdomen as the bowel everts itself outward. This complication is most commonly seen with transverse loop colostomies. |

| Sigmoid colostomy | The most common type of ostomy surgery in which the end of the descending or sigmoid colon is brought to the surface of the abdomen. It is usually located on the lower left side of the abdomen. |
|---|---|
| Skin barriers | Products such as pastes and powders that some people with ostomies used to protect the skin around their stoma before attaching their appliance. The faceplate is also considered to be a barrier as it protects the skin from contact effluent. |
| Stoma | The part of ostomy on the exterior of one's abdomen where the body wastes exits. |
| Temporary colostomy | Allows the lower portion of the colon to rest or heal. It may have one or two openings. |
| Transverse colostomy | The surgical opening created in the transverse colon resulting in one or two openings. It is located in the upper abdomen, middle or right side. |
| Two-piece pouching system | It consists of a separate pouch and faceplate that comprise the Ostomy appliance. |
| Ulcerative colitis | One form of inflammatory bowel disease targeting the colon and affecting its inner lining. |
| Urinary pouching systems | Urostomates can use either one or two piece systems. However, these systems also contain a special valve or spout which adapts to either a leg bag or to a night drain tube connecting to a special drainable bag or bottle. |

## ■ BIBLIOGRAPHY

1. Glossary of terms http://www.dansac.com/en-gb/glossary
2. http://healthyskincaretips.org/skin-care/what-is-karaya-origins-and-uses-of-karaya-gum-in-ostomy-supplies-2/
3. http://www.alcare.co.jp/e/user/product/stoma/glossary/index.shtml
4. http://www.hollister.com/en/ostomycare/ostomycarelearningcenter/ostomyglossary
5. http://www.stomawise.co.uk/types-of-stoma/terminology
6. Ostomy Care and Management: Registered Nurses' Association of Ontario. (2009), Toronto, Canada.
   http://rnao.ca/sites/rnao-ca/files/Ostomy_Care__Management.pdf
7. Ostomy - Stoma - Ostomy Terminology - Ostomy Dictionary
   http://www.ostomysoftware.com/Terminology.html

# Index

Page numbers followed by *f* refer to figure, *fc* refer to flowchart, and *t* refer to table.

## A

Abdomen 55*f*
    four quadrants of 61*f*
Abdominal contours 81
Abdominal distension 123
Abdominal radiation 117
Abdominal wall, anterior 6
Abdominoperineal resection 32, 85
Abscess 137
Accident injury 66
Adhesions 172
Alcohol 164
Allergic skin reactions 130
Amazing ostomates 158
Anorectal
    anomalies 43
    incontinence 42, 49
Antacids 109
    containing magnesium 122
Antibiotics 109
Anti-reflux valve 172
Anus 17
    defunctioning of 84
Atonic colon 31
Australian Council of Stoma
    Associations 156, 157
Azathioprine 135

## B

Baby with colostomy bag 64*f*
Benzoyl peroxide, solution of 135
Bile salt pool 21
Bismuth subgallate 122
Bladder 52
    cancer of 43, 52
    exstrophy of 43, 53
Bleeding and peristomal varices 141
Blowhole transverse colostomy 91

Bowel
    after excision, defunctioning of 84
    defunctioning of 84
    function, normal 116
    ischemia 30, 42, 47, 48, 48*f*
    obstruction 84*f*
Braided sutures 129
Brussel sprouts 163
Burns 85

## C

Candida albicans 134
Caput medusa 138, 139*f*
Carbohydrates 21
    undigested 121
Carcinoma 30
Cecostomy 32, 33, 37
Chlorophyllin copper (derifil) complex 122
Cloacal exstrophy 43
Colchicine 135
Colectomy 172
    subtotal 32, 84
Colitis
    acute 84
    chronic 84
    diversion 142
Colon 19, 48*f*
    carcinoma of 47
    inflammation of inner lining of 45*f*
    injury 84
    resection 93*f*
Colonic cancer 42
Colonic conduit 32, 37
Colonic inertia 85
Colonic obstruction 42, 47
Colorectal cancer 84
    incidence of 1
Colorectal malignancy 47
Colorectal polyps 44*f*

Colostomy 22, 32, 35*f*, 57, 71, 84, 85,
    109, 172
    ascending 32, 32*f*, 33*f*, 37, 59, 172
    Association 156
    completed loop 28
    descending 34, 34*f*, 37, 58, 60, 61*f*, 116
    distal colostomy 24
    double barrel 29, 29*f*
    general 22
    indications for 87*t*
    irrigation 11, 116
        principles of 117
    left transverse 58
    middle colostomy 23
    nonfunctioning 133*f*
    permanent 179
    proximal colostomy 23
    right transverse 58
    sigmoid 32*t*, 34, 37, 57, 59*f*, 61*f*, 116, 180
    temporary 117, 180
    transverse 32, 32*t*, 33*f*, 34, 37, 59*f*,
        60, 61*f*, 180
Congenital disease conditions 44
Constipation 85, 142
    management of 125
    prevention of 125
    relief 106, 124
Contraceptives 109
Contracted bladder 43
Convexity 173
Cramping pain, severe 123
Crohn's colitis 84
Crohn's disease 30, 31, 41, 46, 46*f*, 83, 84,
    169, 174
Cut-to-fit pouch 77
Cystic fibrosis 67

### D

Dapsone 135
Davol product-made out of gum rubber 10
Decubitus ulcers 85
Diarrhea 19, 85, 142, 171
    management of 122
    stomal 142
Diet, influence of 19
Dietary and fluid modification 124
Digestion, complete process of 17
Digestive system
    different parts of 17
    works 16
Disease, excision of 84

Distal ileum, division of 90*f*
Diuretics 109
Diverticular disease 30, 42, 45, 83, 84
Diverticulitis 174
Diverting loop colostomy, completion
    of 29*f*
Drug
    excretion 130
    interactions 130

### E

Ectopia vesicae 50
Eczema 130
Effluent under pouching system,
    leakage of 134
Electrolytes 122
Embolus 48
End colostomy 38, 84, 86, 87, 101*f*
End ileostomy 39, 84, 85, 88, 88*f*, 101
    formation of 90*f*
End ostomy construction 174
Enterostomal nurse, role of 97
Enterostomal Therapists Nursing
        Education Program 7
Enterostomal therapy 100
    nurses 145, 151, 175
Esophagostomy 37
Esophagus 17

### F

Faceplate 175
Familial adenomatous polyposis 44, 175
Familial polyposis coli 41
Fascial defect 140
Fascial support, lack of 140
Fat malabsorption 21
Fecal diversion 85*t*, 127
Fecal incontinence 30, 84
Fecal pouch, application of one-piece 77
Feeding tube, placement of 41*f*
Fistula 85, 130, 134
    peristomal 136
Fluid
    and electrolyte balance 24
    components 122
Fluid-electrolyte imbalance
    management of 123
    prevention of 123
    signs of 122
    symptoms of 122

Folliculitis 134, 175
Food
    blockage, recognition and
        management of 123
    intolerance 122
Fungal Candida albicans 136


## G

Gas
    and odor, control of 121
    forming foods 121
    producing 106, 124
Gastric juice 19
Gastrointestinal
    function 30
    secretions 18*f*
    tract 20*f*, 130
Gastrostomy 37
Gold coast ostomy association 156
Granuloma 133*f*
    peristomal 133*f*


## H

Handicapped ostomates, challenges
        faced by 150
Hartmann's procedure 27, 28*f*, 32, 38, 176
Healthy stoma 101*f*, 105*f*
Hereditary disorder 175
Hereditary non-polyposis colorectal
        cancer 41, 44
Hernia 136*f*
    parastomal 136*f*
    peristomal 116
Herniation, internal 139
Hirschsprung's disease 30, 43, 65, 66*f*
Human digestive system, parts and
        functions 16*f*
Hydrocolloid 137
Hydrocolloid skin barriers 8
Hygiene, poor 130
Hyperplasia, severe 137
Hypertension, portal 138
Hypovolemia 21


## I

Ileal conduit 32, 39, 53, 177
    stoma creation 54*f*
Ileal pouch anal anastomosis 22

Ileal resection 19
Ileal urinary conduit 161
Ileo anal
    anastomosis 32
    pouch procedure 84
Ileostomates 21
Ileostomy 31, 37, 38, 59*f*, 60, 61*f*, 84, 88,
        109, 123, 131, 177
    construction 22
    continent 173
    functioning 133*f*
    lavage 139
    permanent 161
    pouches 71
    predisposing diseases 31
    well-established 139
Ileum 19
    segment of 42*f*
Imperforate anus 65, 65*f*
Incontinence 85
Inflammatory bowel disease 31, 65, 83, 177
Inflammatory disease
    complications 85
    conditions 45
Inguinal colostomy 6
International Ostomy Association 155, 156
Intestinal consistency 20, 20*f*
Intestinal continuity 94
Intestinal segments 19
Intestine, small 24
Intrauterine device, use of 169
Irradiation damage 30, 49
Irrigating stoma 119*f*
Irrigation 178
Irritant dermatitis 103*f*
Ischemia 131
Ischemic bowel disease 137


## J

Jejunal and ileal absorption, normal 18
Jejunostomy 30, 37
    by Maydl's method 30*f*
Jejunum 19
    resection 19
Joint diseases 150


## K

Karaya 178
    gum 8
Kock pouch 173

### ▪ L

Lactase deficiency 21
Lactobacillus 122
Laparoscopic colostomy 92
Laparoscopic ileostomy 92
    preparation for 93*f*
Laparoscopic instruments, orientation
    of 93*f*
Liver 17
Loop colostomy 27, 36, 42*f*, 84
    closure of 36*f*
    defunctioning of 87
Loop end colostomy 28*f*, 87
Loop ileostomy 37, 42*f*, 84, 89, 91*f*, 101*f*
    ileo-anal pouch 32
Loop ostomy creation 178
Loop stoma 7, 36

### ▪ M

Maydl jejunostomy 30
Meconium ileus 43, 67, 67*f*
Mental handicaps 150
Mental illness 150
Metabolic problems 133
Methotrexate 135
Motor neuron disease 150
Motor sensory illness 150
Mucocutaneous junction 138
Mucocutaneous separation 130, 132
Mucosal implants 140
Mucosal ischemia 131
Mucous fistula 35, 35*f*, 38, 39, 87*f*, 127
Myelomeningocele 50

### ▪ N

Natural yoghurt 163
Nausea 123
Necrosis, stomal 131, 131*f*
Necrotizing enterocolitis 43
Neonatal necrotising enterocolitis 65
Neurogenic bladder 50, 52, 53
Nonadherent gauze 137
Non-steroidal anti-inflammatory
    agents 109
Nystatin topical powder 136

### ▪ O

Obligatory ileal sodium 21

Obstruction
    relief of 84
    severe 50
Obstructive disease condition 47
Obstructive pulmonary disease,
    chronic 130
Odor
    control 106, 124
    prevent 170
    producing 106, 124
Ostomate 108*f*, 152
    bill of rights 127
    diagnosis 149
    for medical advice 149
    groups 152
    physically 121
    troubleshooting foods for 124*t*
Ostomist
    general dietary tips for 163
    with fecal stoma 163
Ostomy 1, 2, 16, 161, 179
    and social media 152
      facebook 152
      twitter 152
      youtube 153
    appliances at display 160
    Association of India 155
    Association of Los Angeles 7
    Associations in India and abroad 155
    bag
      one-piece 72*f*
      two-piece 72*f*
    care 100
      agencies in 154
      development of 13, 14
      terms of 153
    closure and time 96
    double barrel 127
    management 127
      system 55
    permanent 179
    pouches 10*f*
      and accessories 72*f*
    pouching systems 179
    service 154, 155
      development of 155
    surgery 127, 145
    temporary 179
    to student nurses, planning and
      teaching of 145
    travel kit 112*f*

visitor 147, 148
  medical advice 149
  permission 148
  privacy 149
  qualities of 147*f*
  role of 147

### ▦ P

Pancreas 17, 67
Pancreatic juices 19
Panproctocolectomy 32, 84
Paraplegia 85
Parastomal 176
  abscess 134, 135
  hernia 129, 135, 136
Pectin skin barrier 56
Pediatric conditions 43
Pediatric stoma care 64
Peg tube placement 41*f*
Pelvic radiation 117
Pelvic sepsis, severe 169
Pendulous abdomen 58*f*
Peppermint tea 163
Perianal disease 84
Perineal resection, abdominal 38
Peripheral neuropathy 150
Peristomal abscess 130, 134
Peristomal candidiasis 179
Peristomal contact dermatitis
  allergic 179
  irritant 179
Peristomal problems 137
Peristomal skin 136
  irritation 130, 132
    prevention 132
  protection 36
Peristomal skin/plane 179
Peristomal varices 141, 141*f*
Perspiration 130
Plasma sodium concentration 21
Plastic rod 28
Polyposis 44
Poor general health 130
Pouch 54
  after emptying, removing 78*f*
  change, timing of 73
  off in bath 166
  pre-sized 77
  selection criteria and options 81*t*
  sizing of 74
Pouching options 81

Pouching selection 81
Pouching system 56fc, 57*fc*
  part of 175
  procedures 71
  two-piece 180
  types of 71
Predisposing diseases colostomy 30
Proctocolectomy, total 85
Prolapse, stomal 140, 141*f*
Prowess stoma care 154
Psoriasis 104*f*, 130
Pyoderma 135
  gangrenosum 135

### ▦ R

Rectal cancer 42, 84
Rectal fistula 85
Rectal injury 84
Rectus muscle
  sheath 60
  splitting of 90*f*
Rheumatoid arthritis 150

### ▦ S

Saliva, composed of 19
Scars 56
Scelerosing cholangitis, primary 141
Sclerosis, multiple 150
Semi digested food travels 17
Sepsis, resolution of 84
Short chain fatty acids, deficiency of 142
Sigmoid colon, resection of 7
Skin
  barrier 79*f*, 180
  care, routine 143
  complications
    causes 103fc
    management 103*fc*
    types 103fc
  condition 102
  creases 56
  permeability, changes in 130
  preparation-soaps 130
  problems 130
  surrounding stoma, cleaning 78*f*
Small bowel
  disease 84
  stoma 121
  water absorption, determinant of 21

Sodium
  absorption 19
  losses, stomal 21
Sphincter repair 84
Spina bifida 43, 50, 52, 53, 66, 67*f*
Spinal cord
  injury 52
  trauma 50
Split ileostomy 84
Stenosis 130, 138*f*
  sight of 137
  treating mild 137
Steroids 109
Stoma 57, 127, 135, 137, 140, 142, 168, 180
  appliance 8, 105*f*
    key developments in 8
    used 166
  appropriate 132
  bag 112*f*
    children's 69*f*
    infant with 68*f*
  care 12, 64, 68, 149, 153, 160
    evolution of 3
    history of 3
    nurse 162, 170
    websites offering 153
  characteristics 81
  classification of 41
  closure 35
  color of 100
  complications 129, 129*fc*
    type of 129
  concealment of 124
  construct good 121
  construction, methods of 83
  creation 145
    principles of 55
  defunctioning 129
  diverting 41, 42*f*
  drug possible effect on 171
  edema of 133
  end 38
  eversion of 89*f*
  flush 175
  forming surgery 1, 162, 165
  functioning of 145
  good healthy 121
  input 41, 41*f*
  large bowel 121, 123
  locations, desirable 60, 61*f*
  maintenance of 116

  marking, site of 90*f*
  nonfunctioning 127
  nurses, on call 152
  obstructing 106, 124, 140*f*
  output 41, 42*f*
  patient, educating 126
  physiology of 18, 19
  pouch made of plastic bag 11
  presence of 126
  problems in 121
  products, application of 77
  prolapse 116
  retracted 131, 132*f*
  retraction, incidence of 131
  revision 142
  site
    marking of 62*f*
    of abdominal 26
    selection 59
  sitting, poor 130
  spout and size 102
  stricture 137
  support group 152
  surgery 2, 4, 67, 84*t*
    key developments in 4
    principles of 83
  surgical principles of 83
  swelling 123
  temporary 83
  types of 26, 37*t*, 60, 81, 84*t*, 145
Stomal complications 130*t*
Stomal lumen, constriction of 137
Stomal skin
  causes of 134*t*
  complications, causes of 134*t*
  management causes of 134*t*
Stool
  control, loose 124
  increased/loose 124
  malodorous floating 21
Stress incontinence 52*f*
Stroke 150
Surgeon and stoma nurse 147
Surgery
  incidence of 50
  principles of 92
Sweat glands 67
Swelling, stomal 123

■ **T**

Toilet-flushable pouches 10*f*

Transjugular intrahepatic portosystemic
    shunt 138
Transureteroureterostomy 53
Trauma 30, 49, 83-85, 142
    abdominal 3
Travelers' diarrhea 167
Trephine 91
    colostomy procedure 92*f*

## ▣ U

Ulcer 134
    pressure 104*f*
    unroof 134, 137
Ulcerative colitis 31, 41, 45, 66*f*, 84, 161, 180
    stages of 46*f*
Umbilicus 56
Underwent permanent ileostomy 161
United Ostomy Association 7
    America 155
Ureteral anastomosis 95*f*
Ureteral conduit anastomosis
       completed 95*f*
Uretero-colic anastomosis, failed 43
Ureterostomy 37
Uric acid stones 22
Urinary
    bladder to cancer 161
    conduit 50
    diversion 50, 51*f*, 52, 53
    incontinence 43, 53
    pouch, application of one-piece 81
    pouching systems 180
    stoma 1, 53

construction of 51
    pouch system options for 79
stone formation 22
system 43
    normal 50*f*
tract 50
    abnormalities of 52
Urostomy 39, 54, 60, 61*f*, 109, 177
    continent 173
    pouch 53*f*

## ▣ V

Vesicostomy 53
Visual
    deficits 150
    illness 150
Vitamins 109
Volvulus 32, 47, 85
Vomiting 123

## ▣ W

Warfarin 171
World media plays 152
World Ostomy Day 159, 160
Wound ostomy continence nurse, role
    of 151
Wound, Ostomy and Continence
    Nurses Society 156

## ▣ Y

Yeast infection 104*f*

EU GSPR Authorised Reprsentative
Logos Europe, 9 rue Nicolas Poussin
1700, La Rochelle, France
Phone: +33 (0) 6 67 93 73 78
E-mail: contact@logoseurope.eu

www.ingramcontent.com/pod-product-compliance
Lightning Source LLC
Chambersburg PA
CBHW080543220326
41599CB00032B/6340